D1546340

Hustle but Healthy

HUSTLE *but* Healthy

The 5 Pillars of **Sustainable Wellness** and **Weight Loss** for the Busy Woman

ROBYN SHAW

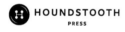

HOUNDSTOOTH
PRESS

COPYRIGHT © 2023 ROBYN SHAW
All rights reserved.

HUSTLE BUT HEALTHY
*The 5 Pillars of Sustainable Wellness and
Weight Loss for the Busy Woman*

FIRST EDITION

ISBN   978-1-5445-3702-3 *Hardcover*
       978-1-5445-3701-6 *Paperback*
       978-1-5445-3703-0 *Ebook*

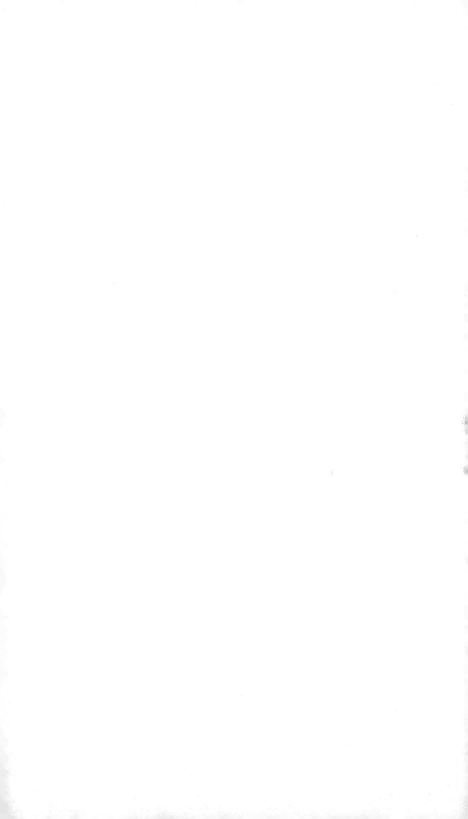

CONTENTS

FOREWORD

I've always believed in balance, but beyond the sense of what we see people preaching all over social media. This is something I honestly feel like I have developed over my thirty years on this planet.

I grew up a very type B personality. Chaotically organized, creative, wildly emotional, and hopelessly and romantically in love with the smallest moments in life, which could make me laugh and cry at the same time. I remember my father coming into my room as a child. He would play the guitar as I fell asleep. I would cry myself to sleep most nights listening to him play. And he would say, "Darling, it's ok. You're an artist. You just feel things more than others do."

For someone who doesn't have the greatest memory, that moment has stuck with me forever. It's like I have a photograph of it burned into my memory.

As I grew up, I fell in love. A lot. Like Taylor Swift, hopelessly, romantically, a lot. I also got my heart broken a lot because when I fell, I fell hard. When I broke, I also shattered. I believe it was with romantic relationships that I truly started to find my pragmatic, rational side, because I was also forced to take a deep, hard look at the relationship I knew the most—my parents'. Being a mediator in my parents' marriage most of my life, I was thrown into looking at relationships a certain way. Without getting into too many details of my personal life right off the bat here, I'll just share that my parents had a complicated relationship. And the closeness I had with my parents left me always feeling obligated to interject myself and help in any way that I could.

I also own a business. And I don't think there's any successful business owner out there who lacks the ability to think rationally and make smart decisions for its growth. All personal emotions aside.

Now, this balance is what makes me, me. The hopeless romantic who wants to travel the world and fall in love, while at the same time investing in her RRSP (Registered Retirement Savings Plan) for a future with her partner. The artist who would love to create beautiful things forever and live in a cabin in the woods but also really values a steady income. The romantic who wants to own a tiny house and travel the country but also realizes the sacrifices that come along with that. The business owner who wants to create a vision bigger than life but also is great at crunching the numbers and making the tough, in-the-moment decisions.

It's benefitted me in so many areas, being:

- flexible and strong
- free and in control
- graceful and powerful
- creative and logical
- carefree and pragmatic

This is the same approach I take with my coaching. Health and wellness are mindset and spiritual, but they're also education and knowledge. It's thinking, but it's also application. It's manifesting, but it's also actionable steps. Not just one thing will ever get you to the ultimate you. You need to learn how to build all the sides of you.

And that's how I want you to view this book moving forward—multifaceted, if you will. This book truly is a piece of me. It's thoughts, ideas, lessons, and information I've compiled over years of coaching and owning BODZii—a seven-figure coaching company that helps busy women lose weight sustainably.

I've been lucky enough to work with women across the globe on their health and weight loss journey. Each and every woman is unique in their own wonderful way, but we share a lot of the struggles we face on our journey to ultimate health, happiness and body confidence. It's a mix of mindset struggles and having the correct and factual information. A mix of navigating our way through a world of misinformation, of doubt and self-sabotage. A health journey is a delicate balance, an art if you will, of understanding ourselves in a crazy world. And it's piecing together a million different pieces into a puzzle that works specifically just for you. I'm here to help you filter through those puzzle pieces and help you quickly and efficiently eliminate ones that don't fit so that you get closer to the best version of yourself.

This book will share stories, quotes, weight loss information, motivational messages, and the best coaching practices. There will be questions, journaling prompts, and the odd exercise for you to do as you read through this book. This book is meant to be read from start to finish, and the ideas and strategies you'll read in this book are meant to be thought about and acted on.

And that is the most important part.

Action.

Because you won't find all the latest studies on weight loss in this book. You aren't going to get all the nutritional science behind how we lose weight. And this definitely isn't a book to give you another new trend or fad diet. I'm not going to tell you to cut things out of your life or diet. I'm not going to tell you to go on a juice cleanse. I'm definitely not going to tell you to take certain supplements to see a new low on the scale. I haven't found the magic pill. I haven't come across some new revelation in weight loss. I'm here to keep it real and give you the truth.

Weight loss does not and will never look the same for everyone. There is a reason why each and every single diet and program out there has results and also failures. Because every diet out there works for some people and doesn't for others. And that is just the hard (and yes, annoying) truth about all of this. I wish I could tell you it's easy.

Where people get caught up in their weight loss journey is never a lack of information. Google "how to lose weight" and you'll get about 1,130,000,000 results in 0.68 seconds. That's over one billion puzzle pieces you have to work through. It's a reason why people get caught up in the execution.

This book will give you the information you need to execute consistently and with confidence through your health and weight loss journey, especially as a busy woman. Because let's face it. you have a lot on your plate, and you don't have the time or patience anymore for another failed attempt at discovering your best self.

As you start this book, I have something I want to give you. And this is your very first step in taking action. The first five days of you reading this book are going to be paired with five days of workouts, mindfulness activities, and meals I want you to follow. There's no time like the present to jump in. So type the link below into your web browser and access your e-book right now! www.bodzii.com/5-healthy-days.

INTRODUCTION

Hustle, but also Drink Water and Sleep and Stuff

Hustle but healthy has been a bit of a tagline that I've been using in my coaching practice and business for a few years now. I'll tell you why.

First off, it's catchy as hell.

Second, as a BODZii member, we hustle. But hold on now...

Get that early millennial, Wolf of Wall Street, no sleep, all work, no play image out of your mind. That's not what hustle means anymore. Not in our world, anyway. Hustle means that you work hard in your career, you're a busy mom, you have a family to take care of, and you're running to business meetings, appointments, and social outings. You care about what you do, and you tend to prioritize a lot of things ahead of yourself. And maybe you're not running yourself into the ground, per se, but you sure aren't putting yourself first amongst all the other things you have going on.

Trust me, I know what that feels like.

Now, I don't have a family or kids (do fur babies count?) that I need to take care of, but I put a lot of pressure on myself to be successful at whatever I do. My business, my coaching practice, that's my baby. And every single day I have to work hard at making sure that I'm putting myself first. Because if I don't show up, my business suffers. My clients suffer. You suffer. This book may have never been a thing if I had not recognized early on that the only way I can get to where I want to be is if I'm showing up every single day. And the only way I can show up every single day is if I'm taking care of myself.

You, the career-driven woman, the mother, the best friend, the wife, the girlfriend, the employee, the business owner, the daughter—we all have something in common. We are all busy. And we are all the curators of our own life. You hustle because you want more for yourself, and you want to be good at what you do. You want to be a good mother, a good friend, and a good employee. You care, and that's why you work hard.

These are the same reasons why it can be especially difficult for you to navigate and execute a successful health and weight loss plan. It might seem like this is an area that's missing in your life. You have it together in a lot of ways and in a lot of areas, but this seems to be one thing you just can't figure out. And that's why this is so hard—because you're so short on time already, the thought of putting time and effort into something that won't end up working for you and getting you results...well, you're not about to do that. I get it.

On top of that, you have this belief that if you can't go all in, there's no point, right?

We need to spend hours in the gym, hours meal prepping,

tracking every single thing we eat forever! Actually...no. That overwhelming thought is exactly the thing that's paralyzing you from moving forward.

So what does hustle but healthy mean?

It means that you see prioritizing you and your health as your responsibility as a busy woman. You want to be there as the absolute best version for your kids, your partner, and your career. You use self-care, fitness, and proper nutrition as a way to show up for the things that are important to you. And most importantly, you're balancing it all.

This is exactly the place we're going to work on getting you to. You're no longer stressed about working out; you fit it in. You're not worried about what you're going to make for dinner when you get home from work; it's already figured out. You're not yo-yoing between diets and attempts to shed pounds; you're embracing the journey and living the healthy lifestyle you've always wanted.

That, my girl, is what hustle but healthy means.

Let's get into what exactly this book is going to lay out for you.

As mentioned, there are a few things along a health and weight loss journey that we all share. Many (like many, many) things are very different for each individual. This makes it impossible for me, or anyone, to write a book that is going to give you exactly what you need in every single aspect. However, I can and will tell you the exact building blocks that every single busy woman needs if they're looking for sustainable weight loss.

Because let's be real. I can get you to lose weight. Fast. So can the next coach. And chances are, if you're reading this book, you've lost weight before. But it didn't stick. And maybe you lost weight a second, third, or even fourth time. But again, none of those times stuck. So weight loss actually isn't the real problem here for a lot of us. Sustainable weight loss is.

And sustainable weight loss is really what we all set out to achieve in the beginning, and it's truly what we all want. But we neglect to adopt the habits, develop the proper mindset, and learn the strategies needed to turn it into a lifestyle. And instead, we get so caught up in the result. Whether for a wedding, a birthday, to fit into a pair of pants—all we want is to see that number on the scale. We get so caught up in it that we don't do the really hard work—how to make it last.

So what is it about sustaining weight loss that is so difficult?

I can break it down into five reasons. And these will be the same five topics we dive into over the course of this book to give you the thoughts and tools you need to overcome these obstacles, create a plan of action, and achieve every single goal you ever set for yourself in the future. And yes, I actually mean that.

You've come here for the weight loss strategies, and don't worry, you'll learn them. But this book can change your life if you let it. How? Because the things you learn about yourself along this journey can be applied to so many other important areas in your life. Having your dream career, finding and building a loving relationship, being the best mom you can be—all these things are big undertakings. And they all require a solid plan of action paired with consistent execution in order to achieve them.

Now let's break down why sustainable results are so difficult.

First, we neglect the most important but very often overlooked part of success—your mindset. Your mind can make or break your success. It's the most powerful tool and probably the most crucial one if you want to make your results last. This journey is full of ups and downs and yes, patience is important, but belief in yourself and your future is even more important. And along the way you'll lose sight of why you started this journey in the first place if you're not working on developing and maintaining a growth mindset. In this section of the book, we'll dive into what a growth mindset looks like and how it applies to your journey. We'll also talk about how we can establish our "whys." Why is it important for you to lose this weight? Why is it important for you to be healthier? To work on yourself? Let's dig deep and create the motivation you need to keep going.

Second, we're much better at planning than we are at executing. Yes, planning is important, but executing is even more important. Knowledge isn't power. Implemented knowledge is. The toughest part about all of this is creating a plan that we can actually stick to. And we'll dive into exactly how you can create this for yourself and move forward with the confidence that you're actually on the right path. We'll talk about:

- inclusive versus reactive goal setting
- how to properly goal map
- creating habits
- and creating your daily nonnegotiables

Third, if and when we do create a plan, we forget about incorporating the most basic habits that lay the foundation for sustainable weight loss. In this section of the book, I'm going to show you the pyramid that my coaches and I have been using to guide our clients to success for over five years. As we know, the base of the pyramid lays the foundation. This is also the section we tend to want to skip for the sake of seeing quicker results. Sleep, stress management, proper hydration, movement, food quality, and building a great relationship with food are all things we'll cover in this section.

Fourth, we get impatient and don't trust the process. Trusting the process is being able to take a big step back and take a macro point of view of your journey. It's common for us to get so consumed by the day-to-day that we forget to look at how far we've come. We eat a slice (or four) of pizza, and we sabotage our entire weekend. We see a number on a scale we don't like, and we get into "screw it" mode. We don't fit into a pair of jeans we hoped to after ten days and want to give up. All of these are examples of us getting too focused on single events. In this section of the book, we're going to talk about the importance of objective data in your health journey and exactly what things you need to measure and track regularly.

Last, we don't build a life raft. This means that we don't build an environment around us that supports our results. This may be one of the hardest things to overcome. Because building a life raft means surrounding yourself with people who have similar goals and aspirations as yours. For me, this is a huge reason why I pay significant money every single month to be a part of a community that's filled with entrepreneurs running multiple seven-figure businesses. We all have similar lifestyles and similar goals, and being surrounded by them every day keeps me focused on my goals. This is also why I attend group CrossFit classes. I'm surrounded by others who are working just as hard as I am. This part can be so challenging because maybe we have friends or family who aren't exactly lining up with our goals. Or maybe we have a job that clashes with a lot of the habits we're trying to create. In this section of the book, we'll talk about how we can manage all of this to make sure every aspect of your life will support you along your journey.

Now, that was a lot of what we don't do well. Flip it the other way around and here's the next five sections of the book:

1. **Get your head right:** how to use a growth mindset to get rid of self-sabotage, gain consistency, and find true self-love.
2. **Plan and execute:** stop the vicious pattern of researching and planning without actually following through.
3. **From the ground up:** using habit stacking and nonnegotiables as the rocks to sustainable weight loss.
4. **Trust the process:** take a step back and learn how to use objective data to measure your progress.
5. **Build your life raft:** surround yourself with people and an environment that will support your journey.

Before moving on, I feel it necessary to say that this book is written for those who are truly looking for lifelong results. This isn't a quick-fix book. This book will not have you losing forty pounds by the time you're done reading it. If you implement the habits and strategies in this book, you'll find yourself:

- having a better relationship with food
- with the most confidence in yourself and your journey ever
- in a better relationship with your weight loss journey
- with way more energy

- prioritizing sleep and stress management
- eating more, better quality food than ever
- moving regularly
- understanding how to edit your lifestyle based on your ever-changing goals

So let's get started.

Section 1

GET YOUR HEAD RIGHT

"Success is the ability to go from one failure to another with no loss of enthusiasm."

— WINSTON CHURCHILL

WHAT IS MINDSET?

The way we think about our journey is how we're going to act throughout it. As we get into this chapter, some of this might be review to you. There may be things you read that you've already read before. And that's a good thing. Because I want you to actually come back to this chapter again and again. Read and reread. Act and act again.

When you think about mindset work, you might think about meditation or sitting in a quiet room with your thoughts. If you're anything like me, you never really saw the value of doing mindset work; you didn't really think, you just acted. And if something was bothering you, you'd accept it for what it was and just keep moving forward. If you're anything like me, you've seen mindset work as a bit "woo woo," or even as a waste of time. Why do mindset work when you can be checking things off your to-do list? That's a question I still, to this day, ask myself regularly.

Well, here's the answer.

Doing mindset work gives you the ability to do everything you do with more intention, more grace, more thoughtfulness, and more success. Doing mindset work allows you to see every obstacle as an opportunity instead of a frustration.

An important word there is intention. Because when you have more intention in your life, you don't just go through the motions, you embrace each moment. And that's something I want you to approach mindset work with—intention.

What's more important is not how often you do mindset work, but how much belief and intention are behind each time.

Here's what I mean by this...

Have you ever been in trouble at school and were made to write lines? I've been there. Don't ask why because honestly, I don't remember what I did, but it must have been passing notes in class or talking while the teacher was talking. Having friends in my classes was always a distraction for me. Anyway, after school I had to sit down and write one hundred times:

"I will not talk while the teacher is talking."

"I will not talk while the teacher is talking."

"I will not talk while the teacher is talking."

"I will not talk while the teacher is talking."

"I will not talk while the teacher is talking."

And no, I couldn't just copy and paste it like I just did here. Handwritten, pencil to paper, one hundred times. Now, in grade six, my mind was *not* taking in the words that I was writing down. My mind was on the fact that this stupid punishment was taking me away from hanging out with my friends after school. Yes, just like your mindset work might seem like valuable time taken away from responding to emails or cooking dinner. Starting to see where I'm going here?

Because I was rushing through the words, making a mess of my lines just so I could get out of there, I really didn't learn a lesson. In fact, I interrupted the teacher the next day and she straight up asked me in front of the class if I had learned anything at all the day before.

I hadn't.

And she made me write one hundred lines again.

Because the repetition isn't what matters. The intention behind it is.

If the teacher had told me to write down the line five times instead of a hundred, but after each line give me five minutes to think about why it's important that I don't do this again, each line would have been way more effective. I probably would have learned my lesson and not interrupted the teacher the next day. And if I had created some intention the first time I wrote the hundred lines, I would have ultimately saved time in the long run—something I was trying to do when I was rushing through each line. You can see how that didn't pay off for me.

And that's exactly how I've lived most of my life. It's taken me about thirty years to get to a point where I can see the immediate effect of doing mindset work because I know how to approach it: with intention.

TYPES OF MINDSET WORK

So above and beyond sitting in a quiet room with your thoughts, what other things would be considered "mindset work"?

- meditation
- yoga or stretching
- journaling
- podcasts
- breathwork

Any one of these options is an amazing way to get the benefits of what mindset work has to offer. And that's building a growth mindset.

MEDITATION

What is meditation? One of my favourite apps, Headspace, can tell you exactly what meditation *isn't!*

> Meditation isn't about becoming a different person, a new person, or even a better person. It's about training in awareness and getting a healthy sense of perspective. You're not trying to turn off your thoughts or feelings. You're learning to observe them without judgment. And eventually, you may start to better understand them as well.[1]

Meditation is being able to sit with no distractions and be present with your thoughts on a journey to creating more mindfulness—the ability to be present, to be fully engaged with whatever you're doing in the moment.

The nice thing about mediation is how versatile it is. You don't just have to sit in absolute silence, left to your own thoughts. That can be scary for a lot of people, myself included. Because what the heck are you supposed to do? Nap?

Guided versus Unguided Meditation

Guided meditation is where you can work with a teacher, or a guide, to help bring you through each practice. This is where apps can come in super handy because you'll be told exactly how to approach each session.

> Most guided meditations follow a similar format: the teacher explains how the mind behaves during meditation, leads you through a particular meditation technique, and then suggests how to integrate this technique into your everyday life.[2]

Calming versus Insight Meditation

The intention for each session and what you walk away with can also vary. And it doesn't always have to be one or the other. Maybe you're looking to relax the mind, focus on the breath, and stop your mind from spinning. Or maybe you're looking to learn something about yourself and the journey you're on and walk away with a lesson.

> People who practice insight meditation often set an intention to transform their minds by developing qualities such as wisdom and compassion. Insight meditation involves focusing on the breath and

being aware of and noting all the physical and mental sensations that arise.[3]

Here are all the forms of mediation and what they have to offer, according to Headspace.com.

Focused attention: This form of meditation is fairly straightforward because it uses the object of our breath to focus attention, to anchor the mind, and maintain awareness. Notice your mind starting to wander? Simply return to the breath.

Body scan: Often, our body is doing one thing while our mind is elsewhere. This technique is designed to sync body and mind by performing a mental scan, from the top of the head to the end of your toes. I like to imagine a glowing ball that starts at the tip of my toes and slowly works its way up to the top of my head until it's floating right above me, like the sun.

Noting: This technique involves specifically "noting" what's distracting the mind. The point isn't to do anything other than draw awareness to thoughts. We "note" the thought or feeling to restore awareness and to learn more about our thought patterns and tendencies.

Visualization: This type of meditation invites you to picture something or someone in your mind; we are essentially replacing the breath with a mental image as the object of focus. It can feel challenging to some, but it's really no different than vividly recalling the face of an old friend naturally, without effort. Visualization can be a very powerful tool for athletes and entrepreneurs.

Loving-kindness: This type of meditation is where we direct positive energy and goodwill first to ourselves, and then to others, which helps us let go of unhappy feelings we may be experiencing. This is a fantastic way to exude gratitude and happiness toward ourselves and other people, especially if we have negative feelings toward someone.

Resting awareness: Rather than focusing on the breath or a visualization, this technique involves letting the mind truly rest. As thoughts enter, you allow them to just drift away instead of distracting you from your practice.

Reflection: This technique invites you to ask yourself a question: perhaps something such as, "What are you most grateful for?" Be aware of the feelings, not the thoughts, that arise when you focus on the question.

YOGA/STRETCHING

Yoga and stretching can be another amazing way to practise mindfulness and give you an opportunity to connect with your body and mind. Personally, what I get from yoga is patience. And that patience I can take with me in my business, my relationships, and my personal growth.

After eight years of coaching and training CrossFit, my brain has become used to high intensity and fast-paced movement. Having patience was definitely not a priority, especially when the point of a workout is to race against the clock. After taking up my yoga practice, all of a sudden my instructor is telling me to hold positions, breathe into the stretch, and flow into a new asana (pose). I had to learn very quickly to be patient and embrace the process because if I didn't, I'd be frustrated and would just want to quit. I'd get nothing out of the session if I wasn't patient.

Yoga is described as a "state of connection and a body of techniques that allow us to connect to anything."[4] As described by Dr. Swami Shankardev Saraswati, yoga is a state of connection and a body of techniques that allow us to connect to anything.[5] And if I were to take anything away from that, it would be the word "connect"

The slow nature of yoga and stretching also forces you to take a beat and slow down. And that itself can be seen as a form of meditation. You can be with your thoughts, you can be with your body.

JOURNALING

Journaling has to be one of my favourite ways to practise mindset development. It's accessible, it can be a daily practice, and it can take as little as five minutes. Talk about being efficient for a busy gal like yourself. And so, if you're looking to bring mindset work into your world for the first time, I would definitely suggest journaling to start.

Here are a couple ways you can begin:

Emotional Dump

An emotional dump is literally writing out all the emotions you have pent up inside of you. Positive, negative, neutral, feelings, emotions, thoughts, all of it! It can be two minutes or fifteen minutes. Go until you feel like you have nothing else to say. I promise you this can be one of the most cathartic things you do in a day. And if you do it in the morning, it starts your day off with a clean slate.

Affirmations and Gratitude Journaling

This is a super quick exercise you can do where you write out a daily affirmation followed by three to five things that you're grateful for. Personally, I believe your affirmation should be the same thing every day. That way you set a clear intention and "keep your eyes on the prize," if you will, daily.

Future Journaling

Set your timer for two to thirty minutes and start writing, in present tense, what your future looks like one year from now. You can write about a specific moment in time, or you can write about how your whole life has changed. Personally, I like to write about a specific moment in time. I envision myself almost frozen in a moment and I write about all the little details. How I'm feeling, what I'm wearing, who's around me, what I'm about to do, and what I've just finished doing. If this is difficult, start by generally writing about what's going on in your life.

When future journaling, it's important to be mindful of what emotions come up as you're writing these details down. If, when you're going through the details of your future, you feel doubt, uncertainty, maybe disbelief, then you should be doing this practice more often until you start to feel hope, excitement, and anticipation.

The point here is to really BELIEVE that this future is yours and that you will get there.

PODCASTS

If you're really having a hard time getting into this whole mindset thing, don't worry. You may know by this point that taking action is so much more important than knowledge. And so, if after reading all these different methods of mindset work, you take zero action, then I've failed!

Podcasts are one of the easiest forms of meditation for action because all you need to do is pop your earbuds in and listen. Make me a promise though and go on a walk, a hike, or sit comfortably when listening. This is your dedicated mindset time, so try your best to eliminate distractions. This, however, might be one of the times I'll let you cook or clean while listening so you can get that multitasking in.

There are so many podcasts out there these days on building a growth mindset, self-development, and personal growth. Here are just a few to get you started:

The Mindset Mentor

Daily Mind Medicine

The Growth Mindset Podcast

The Hustle But Healthy Podcast

Breathwork is a form of meditation that bypasses the mind and forces you into a deeper level of awareness faster than "normal" meditation. As Gwen Dittmar of lifestyle media brand mindbodygreen says, "The practice gives the brain's executive functioning something to focus on, so you can bypass the mental level of consciousness and drop into a deeper state of consciousness."[6]

People might choose to do breathwork instead of meditation because they're looking for more immediate relief from high stress or tension. And the nature of breathwork almost forces you into that state quickly.

Gwen Dittmar also says:

> Meditation is a slow and steady practice that over a period of time will shift our perspective. But many people are seeking relief now, and meditation does not bring the relief they are looking for. Breathwork, on the other hand, can be easier to drop into when you are seeking more immediate feedback. It's a great tool to pull out when you're feeling stressed, overwhelmed, or off-center.[7]

There are many types of breathwork, just as there are many types of meditation. I would recommend finding a guided breathwork video for your first time before practising on your own.

To learn more about breathing techniques, here are a couple of websites for you to visit:

https://www.wimhofmethod.com

pausebreathwork.com

I want you to really go all in on one of these practices as you go through this book. Every time you pick this book up, set a timer for ten minutes and complete a journaling session, a guided meditation, stretching, a breathwork session, or part of a podcast. Put yourself in that calming and focused mindset so that you can come into this book with intention and a clear vision of what you want to take away from it!

YOUR MIND'S ROLE IN SUSTAINABLE WEIGHT LOSS

We've talked lots about what mindset means, but how does this play a role in our journey to health, happiness, and weight loss? First, we can start by talking about a growth mindset and how it will lead us to success.

So what is a growth mindset anyway?

Have you ever thought to yourself, *This is just the way I am, I'm never going to be able to get there*? Have you ever been stuck in a plateau for days or weeks and given up on your plan because it got hard? Do you find yourself wanting something different, achieving new things, but have a really hard time doing the actions it takes to get you there? If there's one thing we know, it's that if you want to be something different, you must do something different.

Enter the growth mindset. And enter Carol Dweck, one of the world's leading researchers on motivation and mindsets:

Why waste time proving over and over how great you are, when you could be getting better? Why hide deficiencies instead of overcoming them? Why look for friends or a partner who will just shore up your self-esteem instead of ones who will also challenge you to grow? And why seek out the tried and true, instead of experiences that will stretch you? The passion for stretching yourself and sticking to it, even (or especially) when it's not going well, is the hallmark of the growth mindset. This is the mindset that allows people to thrive during some of the most challenging times in their lives.[8]

I have this and another quote stuck on my wall in my office that my mentor once said to me. The other one reads, "The size of your business is dependent on the size of the storm you can weather."

The growth mindset is freedom. This is where we persevere in the face of failure. We find inspiration in the success of others. We embrace challenges, accept criticism. We have a desire to learn, to build abilities. And it's the sad and frustrating truth that nine times out of ten, the biggest reason why women, and especially busy women, will not achieve their health and weight loss goals is because of impatience and self-sabotage. It's because we're afraid of challenges; we give up easily. Maybe we're paralyzed by all the information out there on weight loss, realize how much we don't know, and get overwhelmed. These are all traits of a fixed mindset.

A fixed mindset is the idea that we're born one way. The idea that we are who we are, and we have to play with the cards we were dealt. You can see how this state of mind can be a massive thirty-foot-high concrete wall obstacle when it comes to achieving almost anything that lives outside of our comfort zone. Even if that thing is actually just on the other side of a glass wall...

with a door...that's unlocked. The fact that you believe you are "meant to be exactly where you are" can prevent you from ever opening that door.

And that's a paralyzing belief. Yet it's a reality for a lot of us.

When you live with a fixed mindset, you might:

- ignore feedback from others
- shy away from coaching or learning opportunities
- feel threatened by others' successes and think less of yourself
- think that effort is fruitless and a waste of energy
- avoid challenges

I want to be clear in saying that you may have a growth mindset in some areas but a fixed mindset in others. And so even if you resonated with one of those statements above but not all of them, that's still an *opportunity* for you to work on.

See what happened there? Identifying with something negative isn't a negative thing. It's an opportunity.

I also want to share with you that still, to this day, as I'm writing this book as the so-called "expert," I have a fixed mindset when it comes to certain areas in my business and relationships. So trust me when I say that building your growth mindset takes time, patience, and gratitude. And when you feel like you've expanded your mind and limits, you're going to find another more complex area in your life that still needs a little push.

That is something you earn.

One of my business mentors told me once that being a business owner is all about solving problems. And he said that you must earn your right to have high level problems. Because every time you fix a problem in your business, you unlock a higher-level, more complicated one that, once solved, will take you even further. I see so many similarities in health and business the more my business grows. This is just one example. The deeper you get into your health and weight loss journey, the more problems you're going to face, the more plateaus you're going to have, the less the scale is going to move, and the less "WOW!" progress you're going to see.

Of course, we can't lose weight forever. And the more weight we have to lose, the more "WOW!" our progress is going to be in the beginning stages. And so, if you're not putting in the hard work early on in building this growth mindset, your journey...well, it's going to be miserably frustrating. To say the least.

Now, on top of it all, you have a butt load on your plate. Yes, a butt load. It's my book, I can say what I want. And because you're busy running around making the world a better place, being a rockstar mom or an A-Team employee, you also are in this mindset that you just don't have the time to prioritize you. And that, my dear, is just another belief holding you back from being your absolute best self.

"If you want something done, ask a busy person."

— BENJAMIN FRANKLIN

"The more we do, the more we can do; the more busy we are, the more leisure we have."

— WILLIAM HAZLITT

These are two of my favourite quotes when it comes to perceiving busyness. Because it's so damn TRUE! Every single busy woman who has come into our coaching program has been able to find time in their schedule to work out, make food, do mindset work, and to prioritize herself. Every single one. That's because every single woman who comes into the program goes through mindset training—just like we're talking about right now—so they can view their busy schedule as opportunity, not overwhelm. To view their workouts as a responsibility, not an inconvenience. To see their mindset work as a necessity, not a waste of time.

The way you approach something will always determine the outcome. You have 100 percent control over the energy you bring to any situation.

Now, let's pause for a moment and put this into practise.

FUTURE JOURNALING EXERCISE

Now that we've covered some good ground on the importance of mindset work in our health and weight loss journey, let's put it into practise.

We've talked about future journaling already. So here's an exercise that I like to do often with my clients.

- Step 1: Get yourself a cute little journal. I mean, a piece of paper will do just fine as well, but a cute journal is always nice.
- Step 2: Set a timer for five to ten minutes.
- Step 3: While the timer is counting down, write out all of the things that could get in the way of you ever reaching your goals. Thoughts, physical things, life events, anything.

> Important: While you're writing, you're going to start to feel some negative emotions. Take note of these and how strongly you're feeling them.

- Step 4: On a scale from 1-10, write down the intensity of the negative emotions that were coming up.
- Step 5: Repeat Step 2.
- Step 6: Let's future journal. While the timer is counting down, write down, in present tense, where you are one year from now. This could be an exact moment in time. This could be a general vision of how your life is different one year from now.

> While you're writing, take note of any positive emotions that are coming up. Hope, excitement, anticipation, or motivation.

- Step 7: On a scale from 1-10, write down the intensity of the positive emotions that were coming up.

Now we get to talk about what this all means. One of your numbers is going to be higher than the other. Likely. Maybe it's not. But we'll figure it all out.

If your negative emotions number is higher than your positive emotions number, it means that you likely let your negative emotion take over and maybe even dictate your actions. When it comes to your health journey, you feel negative emotions more strongly. This could be for a number of reasons. Maybe you don't believe in yourself, maybe you tend to practise some self-sabotage, or maybe you've simply experienced so much frustration and negative emotion in your journey so far that you can't help but have these negative emotions dominate your mind.

If your positive emotions number is higher than your negative, use that. Use that as fuel for your fire. This means that your hope and positive beliefs outweigh the negative. It means that even if frustration, obstacles, and barriers arise, which they will, you're so rooted in your potential future that you won't let them derail you. Being more excited about your future than worried about what could get in the way is what will lead you to act consistently on the path to get there.

Your job is to do this exercise as often, and with as much intention, as needed to increase the gap between your negative and positive number. If, in a few weeks of journaling, your previously higher negative number turns into an equal or even just slightly-lesser-than number, that is a huge win, and you're on your way to approaching your health and weight loss journey with a much more positive state of mind.

As a busy woman, ten to twenty minutes, two to four times a week is all you need to reframe your mindset and to start backing up your actions with a solid mentality. And now's the time to start. Set this book down, whip out your calendar, and schedule in three- to ten-minute journaling sessions over the next seven to ten days.

I'll wait.

WORKING ON YOUR WHY

A huge part of approaching your journey with a positive state of mind is getting a really good handle on why you're embarking on this journey to begin with. And now that you have a good handle on developing and maintaining a growth mindset, let's talk about how we can make it easier on ourselves to stay motivated.

I remember the first time I was told to watch Simon Sinek's "How Great Leaders Inspire Action" video. You might know it better as the "Why" video. You might not have any idea what I'm talking about, in which case, do yourself a solid and put this book down for twenty minutes to catch up.

"The goal is to do business with people who believe what you believe" was a line that stuck with me when I first watched it. And it's definitely stayed with me ever since.

If we think about ourselves as consumers, we assimilate ourselves to brands because we believe what they believe. Or we want people to perceive us as someone who is aligned with a certain brand. The best brands make us act. In this particular case, in the form of buying.

Having a solid "why" acts as a foundation that we can fall back on. As a brand, all actions, systems, messaging, marketing, etc. surround that "why." If the "why" is solid enough, all actions will be aligned, messaging is clear, people are responding positively, and the business is successful.

Now, let's start to look at our individual selves as our own personal brand. Your beliefs, dreams, likes, dislikes, the way you dress, the food you eat, and every action you take every day are building up your personal brand. Just like any other brand, if your "why" isn't solid, your actions have no direction. It's easy to move through life without intention. You put yourself on autopilot and wait for a better moment to take big, intentional action. And it can be really difficult to pull yourself out of this cycle if you're not really familiar with why you want to do something in the first place.

About a year ago, I completely revamped the intake process of our new clients. I was looking at everything from the very first discovery call, the sales call, the initial assessment, right up to their first coaching check-in. Nowhere in any of those four calls did I get a clear understanding of why the client was seeking out a weight loss coach.

Let me back up a little bit though. I *did* ask them why they booked a call with me.

"I want to lose fifteen pounds."

"I want my old jeans to fit again."

"I want to feel good in a bikini."

Now, I don't want to say that these reasons are not valid. They are absolutely, 100 percent valid reasons for wanting to join a program. But are they solid enough to fall back on for the rest of your life as a reason to act a certain way? Will all your actions moving forward align with wanting to lose fifteen pounds? This whole time I was talking about our program as *the* sustainable weight loss program. Our promise was—and still is to this day—designed to be the last coaching program you'll ever need for anything fitness or nutrition related. Yet I was bringing people into the program without knowing what it was that was going to drive them for the rest of their life.

If I was promising people forever results, I needed to evoke forever action. I needed to pull out of them what was going to keep them going. And, well, as we've already discussed, a good "why" evokes action.

So I decided to do some more digging in these initial phone calls. It turned into this process of asking the right questions to get to know someone as best as I could in the time that I had with them.

"Do you have kids?"

"How is your self-confidence?"

"How do you feel when you're eating out in public?"

"What are your relationships like?"

You might be asking yourself, "Uhm, Robyn...what do any of these have to do with me wanting to lose fifteen pounds?"

We're figuring out why you want to lose fifteen pounds. And more importantly, we're figuring out how this "why" is going to impact and drive your actions so you can get to your goal and keep moving forward.

All of a sudden, a goal like:

> My goal is to lose twenty pounds. And I hope that if I can do that, my daughter will see that I'm taking care of myself.

turns into:

> My goal is to be a role model for my daughter. And by doing that, I hope that I'll be able to lose weight in the process.

Notice the big difference there? We've put the driving factors first. We put what matters in your life first. And by doing this, we can align all of our actions with being a good role model for a young girl instead of a number on a scale.

A bit more motivating, don't you think?

In the process of figuring out what your own personal "why" is, we can do a really simple exercise of just asking, "Why do you want to see XYZ result?"

Why do you want to look good in a bikini this summer?

We can change "I want to look good in a bikini so that I feel comfortable at beach parties" to "I want to work on gaining self-confidence, and those actions will result in weight loss."

Why do you want to fit in a pair of jeans?

We can change "I want to fit into my size six jeans again because I feel like I'm aging too quickly" to "I want to feel energized and age gracefully. By doing that, I'll be able to fit into clothes that I love again!"

As you may know by now, I have two major focuses in my life—nutrition and fitness coaching and being an entrepreneur. The similarities between the two become more and more aligned as time goes on. How we can be successful in our personal health and weight loss journey is very similar to how we can be successful in our entrepreneurial journey.

They're both of the same calibre—lasting a lifetime. They both require a level of grit and determination.

They both need a clear WHY, discipline in HOW, and consistency in WHAT.

Find clarity in your **"why"** by putting your values first, as we've already covered. In business, Apple believes in thinking differently. This is their "why." Disney believes in storytelling. And their "why" can be summed up into "we're in the business of telling stories." Apple's is summed in "Think Differently." Your "why" is your beliefs, your values. It's what drives you to stick to your **how**.

Your **"how"** is your actions. This is every action that's going to get you to your goal. It's every decision made, every system followed, and every action followed through that supports your **Why**. Figuring out your goal and then framing it with your why is relatively easy. Where businesses get caught up is not having the discipline to show up every day to execute.

Where weight loss journeys fail is the exact same. We fail to show up, to put in the work, and to make the smallest yet most important decisions. And I know this is likely your missing puzzle piece right now in getting to your "what."

Your **"what"** is your results. And consistent results move you forward. Now, I'm not talking results as just a number on the scale (although that is one example). I'm also talking about the result of getting a great night's sleep. The result of hiring a solid team in a company. As Simon Sinek wrote relating to business, "The only way people will know what you believe is by the things you say and do, and if you're not consistent in the things you say and do, no one will know what you believe."[9] Why is this important in a weight loss journey?

If you have the belief that health is important, and you value your body and its health, yet WHAT you're doing doesn't support that, then your results do not reflect your why. Your **what** does not reflect your **why**. You wake up feeling groggy every morning because you're on four hours of sleep, which is not a reflection of your beliefs.

Now, don't worry. That's exactly why you're here. So that we can connect these three things and get you living in full alignment.

Here's an example of a **why, how,** and **what** that are not in alignment:

WHY: Aging gracefully and maintaining youthfulness.

HOW: Choosing three glasses of wine instead of one; ordering take-out instead of making dinner.

WHAT: Low activity, lethargy, and high body fat percentage.

Here's an example of a why, how, and what that are in full alignment:

WHY: Aging gracefully and maintaining youthfulness.

HOW: Getting to bed before midnight; choosing to get a workout in instead of watch Netflix.

WHAT: Weight loss, tons of life, and energy.

Through alignment of these three things, we can lead a life that we're confident in. We can create a life that we are proud of.

Now it's your turn. It's time to fill out your Why, How, and What.

WHY: Write out why it's important for you to lose weight and work on your health.

HOW: Write out three things you need to execute in order to achieve your goals.

WHAT: Write out the result of doing these three things.

Take it a level up and write these in a journal or on a piece of paper that you can see daily. This is your plan of action in the simplest form possible.

"The way you think, the way you behave, the way you eat, can influence your life by 30 to 50 years."

— DEEPAK CHOPRA

FIND YOUR BALANCE

Mindset is complicated because it includes all our history, our beliefs, and all the thoughts we have about something, which is, in this case, weight loss. A big part of mindset and maintaining a growth mindset, as we've already discussed, is belief. The belief that what you're doing is the right thing for you to be doing, and the belief that you can be and do more than you are right now.

Diet culture has made this very difficult for women. Weight loss and diet culture have constructed nasty beliefs that we need to weigh less, eat less, and take up less space. And slowly along the way it has swept up millions of women and made them believe that they aren't good enough.

Women are smart and resilient, though. Farther down that same road we got fed up with the feeling of unworthiness and decided to take a stand against all the things that made us feel that way. Crash diets, pills, restriction, overexercising, undereating, meal plans, the celery diet, juice cleanses, teatoxes. And rightfully so!

But then this slowly started to turn into anything that fell into the health and wellness category, because anything that fell into this category has caused women so much pain that they want nothing to do with it. Salads, working out, morning routines, and even meditation or journaling are all giving women the same "ick" feeling.

With pain and hurt often comes rebellion against the thing that has caused this pain. When a boyfriend breaks up with us, we are hurt, we are broken. And we often will find someone who's nothing like the man who broke our heart. I remember in high school my rugby-playing, jock, and Mr. Popularity boyfriend and I split up. The next boy I dated was a tattooed, slender musician who had absolutely nothing in common with my previous boyfriend. The point here is that women and diet culture have broken up. And now women have moved on to the thing that's helping them heal.

Self-care and self-acceptance.

With the self-care movement has come an incredible number of women taking the time to prioritize themselves. Finally. But what does self-care really mean? We often see girls on Instagram hash-tagging #selfcare underneath a photo of their most recent Sephora purchase. Maybe you're guilty of this—heading to the salon and taking a "self-care day." Or even more with this rebellion against diet culture, it's not just getting nails done and taking a "me" day. It's turning into ordering a pizza and skipping the gym, getting rid of any routine, and maybe even hanging out in sweats all day for the sake of accepting yourself for where you are and not falling into the traps of diet culture.

Don't get me wrong, I myself love a good Sephora shop, and there are definitely days where I'll crush a pizza to myself. But what are we trying to achieve when we practise these things for the sake of self-care? And why does it seem to be that we keep failing at it?

We do our nails or take a day to ourselves, and it takes our mind off our daily stressors and pain. For the moment, life seems peaceful. And for the moment, we're happy about the way we look and feel. But we're missing the point.

Self-care is any action that we do deliberately in order to increase our mental or physical health. Self-care practised with intention and understanding should help us lead a life of balance and happiness. It shouldn't be an act creating temporary relief that only rushes back once finished. It should be a variety of acts that are practised consistently.

Self-care is the collection of actions we take that lead us to self-love.

So now I should mention that my tattooed musician boyfriend and I didn't work out either. Although he had traits I loved, I also missed traits of my ex. And instead of rebelling so hard in the opposite direction, I needed to find my balance. Of course, hindsight is always 20/20, and I would have never known that without experiencing it. Remember that your pain will always give you the experiences you need to learn about yourself. In this case, true self-care is finding that balance. Health and wellness have hurt you, diet culture has hurt you, but that doesn't mean every element of it is bad. You need to find that balance.

You need to believe in what true self-care and self-love really mean.

I thought I would take this time to give you four ways you can start to look at self-care in a new, more long-term and sustainable way. Because that's what we're all about. And learning how to practise true, sustainable self-care is one of the best ways we can practise a growth mindset.

1. BREAK UP WITH PERFECTIONISM

Self-care and self-love are needed by those of us who work so incredibly hard every day chasing the idea of perfection. The constantly changing, shape shifting, and equivocal notion of perfectionism. It's just as exhausting as it sounds. Working with highly driven people over the past five years, I've been able to see this firsthand.

Most of the time we're too hard on ourselves, always looking back on what we could have done better. This unfortunately leads to a lot of self-criticism, and in some cases self-deprecation. This annoying little voice inside of us that's persistent in telling us that we need to do more is the trademark of perfectionism.

Studies have shown the direct correlation with perfectionism and heightened stress-cortisol levels. We know that chronic stress leads to high blood pressure and hypertension. In slighter cases, it can cause stomach issues, headaches, muscle tension, irritability, poor food choices—the list goes on.

So what can we do to break up with perfectionism and embrace balance, consistency, and continuous progress instead?

Awareness is the first step. Realize that perfectionism isn't setting you up for any success—let alone perfection. Realize that perfectionism is bad for you. And you deserve better.

Constantly picking at your imperfections slowly chips away at your self-worth and ultimately your happiness. And happiness isn't something you deserve or not. You are born with the right to happiness. You are entitled to a happy life. The United Nations even proclaims that March 20 is the International Day of Happiness, and that "the pursuit of happiness is a fundamental human goal."[10] Block it in your calendar!

Of course, changing these habits takes time. It's not something that's going to disappear the next time you look in the mirror or have a less-than-perfect test result. But what we can do is start to realize that each time we feel these emotions is a time for us to practise fighting against them. It's a time for us to better ourselves.

Embrace these moments, for each moment you want to pick yourself apart is also a moment for you to practise self-compassion.

2. CULTIVATE SELF-COMPASSION

Self-compassion requires us to be warm and understanding toward ourselves in a time of inadequacy, failure, or suffering.

Practising self-compassion can help us build strength in the face of adversity, it can help us deal with embarrassment or judgement. It can help us better understand ourselves. Although easier said than done, going easy on ourselves might just be the thing we need sometimes.

I'll be clear in saying that I'm all for discipline and a great work ethic, so long as it doesn't run you to the ground. In the gym, we always say, "choose the rest day before the rest day chooses you," and I find this just as applicable when it comes to self-care and self-compassion.

Make sure you take the time to practise positive self-talk, journaling, meditation, or mindfulness exercises to acquire an abundance of self-compassion that will carry you through your most difficult times.

Dr. Kristin Neff defines self-compassion as a construct that encompasses three components:

- self-kindness (i.e., treating oneself with understanding and forgiveness)
- recognition of one's place in shared humanity (i.e., acknowledgment that people are not perfect and that personal experiences are part of the larger human experience)
- mindfulness (i.e., emotional equanimity and avoidance of overidentification with painful emotions)[11]

It's easy to get overwhelmed with something so elusive, so it's important to make sure we have a plan and practices in place to help us achieve this.

Take a moment today to identify if negative self-talk is something you should be working on, and then take some small steps in moving forward. Every time you find or catch yourself talking negatively about yourself or something you're doing, take note of it. And yes, it can actually be a written note. I don't want you to do anything about it, just note it. In this moment you're not trying to change it or fix it. I just want you to become self-aware of how many times a day this is happening.

3. LEARN ABOUT YOUR BODY

Many times a day I talk to people who aren't happy with their bodies. They want to be thinner, stronger, have more muscle, have clearer skin, or look better in their clothes. We just talk an awful lot about what diet culture has done to us.

But real self-care comes from taking time to educate yourself on how your brain and body work. It's time to improve your body literacy.

What goes on inside your stomach when you eat certain foods?

What's happening in your brain when you have an anxiety attack?

What's happening in your brain when you go for a jog?

What is causing you to have breakouts? Or poor, sleepless nights?

Why are you not fitting in your clothes the way you used to?

Why are you tempted to eat sugary foods so much recently?

All these are completely understandable, frustrating, and valid questions. And they all have answers.

Taking the time to answer some of these questions for yourself will hopefully allow you to understand that the body is an incredibly complex system. The body is also an amazing machine. Infinite combinations of biological and emotional nuances lead our body to change, adapt, and also need certain things.

A simple change in atmosphere and surrounding environment can play a critical role in your body's biochemistry. A change in physical or emotional environment is a stressor which impacts our body in multiple ways. This is because our brain and our nervous, endocrine, and immune systems are constantly interacting.

Why is this important? Because when you come home after a long day at work where your boss yelled at you and you're feeling emotional, it might prevent you from reaching for a pint of ice cream if you understand one important thing.

That the mesolimbic dopaminergic system, a.k.a. "the reward pathway," in your brain is actively pushing you eat highly palatable foods since you're stressed and, that it's not just you "feeling weak" and in need of some comfort food.

The more we can understand, the more we realize the power we carry. The more we understand the pressures we put on our brain and body day in and day out and how precisely they respond, the more reason we have to love and treat our bodies like the temples they are.

4. ASK MORE FROM YOUR BODY

My last point pushes you outside of your comfort zone. Because outside of your comfort zone is where magic happens. Magic being growth, learning, acceptance, self-awareness, and love.

To care and love your body is to allow it to show you what it can do.

Not honouring that is like never enrolling your child into any lessons, classes, or school. You're stripping away potential and preventing any growth.

If you feel like your body is a poor representation of your outgoing, active, vivacious spirit, then get outside on an adventure. Go hiking, climbing, biking, and running with a group of people. Allow your body to thrive and become the manifestation of your energy.

If you're career driven, have lofty goals, and are ready to push forward in the corporate world, don't let your body slow you down. Eat good food, stay hydrated, sleep well, and recover. Allow your body to become the productivity machine it wants to be.

If you know your body can give you more, ask for it. As we've learned, the body is an amazing, complex machine.

The body has run a sub-two-hour marathon, free soloed El Capitan, run 900 kilometers in nine days across the Pyrenees, put 266 kilograms overhead, and swum 140 miles across the Adriatic Sea. It's nothing short of incredible.

How you push your body is up to you, as long as it's a little further than it is now. As long as it's out of your comfort zone. And as long as you thank your body for getting you there. Every time.

Real self-care requires routine, planning, learning, movement, compassion, mindset work, journalling, and thoughtfulness. If we can shift our mindset and beliefs about what self-care is, we can use them along our journey to help us stay consistent, motivated, and happy.

Testimonial from member Renee:

"This is the first time I've ever felt 100 percent at peace with my body. I've always told myself that I had to be a certain size to be happy and accept myself. But I realized that you can be happy along the journey even if you're not yet exactly where you want to be.

I asked myself the other day, *If I don't lose a pound ever again would I be happy with where I am?* And I answered, *YES!*"

Section 2

PREP, VISUALIZE, PLAN, AND EXECUTE

You want so much more for yourself. You have all these visions and you've been working on your mindset. You've been working hard on rewriting all these negative beliefs that decades of diet culture have etched in your mind. And you now finally have your eyes on the prize.

But you just can't seem to piece it together. You can't seem to execute.

It's time to dive into how we can start putting together a plan that we can actually execute. What's important for me in this section is that you find a unique solution to your unique life. Because what's important is you being able to maintain all the roles and responsibilities you have as a busy woman and also having the confidence that you can still execute—even if it is on something small. A small step forward is always better than no step.

UNDERSTANDING WHAT'S AHEAD

There are six elements to a rock-solid journey. And this is where I want to introduce Seth Godin's idea of a Success Hierarchy.[12]

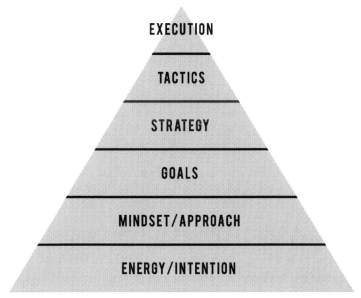

Figure 1

ENERGY AND INTENTION

You are a living energy field. And your body is composed of energy-producing particles, each of which is in constant motion. So, like everything and everyone else in the universe, you are vibrating and creating energy. And whether you believe in positive and negative energy or not, you do create it. And the energy which you bring to a situation will also be the way you react to it.

Attitude, like intention, is the reason why you're doing it at all.

MINDSET AND APPROACH

How are you going to approach your journey? Do you approach things with more of a gut feeling? Do you like finding studies and evidence to back things up? Are you coachable and willing to ask questions? Or are you going to figure things out on your own?

You have the choice to approach your journey with a curious growth mindset, or you can approach your journey with a closed mind. We all have a way we like to do things, but how you approach your journey will dictate your actions and ultimately your outcome.

GOALS

Goals are your vision. They are what drive motivation for most people. If any action is going to happen at all, it's going to be because we got really excited about our goals.

STRATEGY

A strategy is an action plan that you will take in the future to achieve a final, end goal. Strategies help to define your long-term goals and how you go about achieving them.

If someone is trying to reach their goals solely with strategy, they won't get anywhere, since tactics are the concrete action items that take you where you need to go. When a team uses strategy alone, the only thing that they'll be doing is planning to achieve goals instead of doing the work that needs to be done to achieve them.

TACTICS

While strategy is the action plan that takes you where you want to go, the tactics are the individual steps and actions that will get you there. In a weight loss journey context, this means the specific actions you'll take to implement the initiatives outlined in the strategy.

EXECUTION

This is the action you take. Strategy means nothing without tactics, and tactics mean nothing without execution. They're just plans. And the easiest way for a plan to fail is without execution.

Most of us are good at about 50 percent of these things. We set goals, we strategize, we seek out tactics, we research, we read, we save workouts, and we have hundreds of saved Instagram posts with the intention of following through one day.

But we never do.

So why are we so crappy at executing? In every initial call with potential clients I ask the question, "At this moment in your journey, do you feel like you know what it takes to lose weight?" About 80 percent of the time the answer I hear back is, "Yes, I just have a really hard time actually acting on it."

And so this tells us that knowledge really means nothing. Knowledge is not power. Implemented knowledge is power.

I believe that this age of information we live in has stunted our ability to act, to experiment, and to get curious about things. We have everything we could possibly want to know at our fingertips. So why try and figure anything out on our own? We genuinely think the internet can probably tell us more about ourselves than we know. We search "how many calories should I eat in a day?" as if the internet knows the ins and out of our physiology. We google "how do I lose weight?" as if we're about to read our way into shedding body fat.

And after spending the first section of this book talking about energy, intention, mindset, and how we approach our health journey, it's time to move on to how we can set goals that we're actually going to follow through on.

GOAL SETTING

Every so often I'll run a twenty-eight-day nutrition and lifestyle challenge. To say these challenges are successful would be an understatement.

Each day I'll hop on the Facebook group where we share our successes, and I'll get the participants to share a win they had over the weekend. One comment read,

> I don't think my diet is where I want it to be. Mostly because of lack of discipline with Canada day and the holidays. But my biggest achievement in the past two months is giving up sugar almost completely. I went one month and four days without getting anything from Tim Hortons (which was a daily habit), and now I don't feel I need it anymore. Making small sustainable changes like drinking lots of water and cooking my own meals, and they've made a huge difference so far.

On a different day, I was on a run and listening to a Nike Run Club guided run. It started talking to me about doing the things that you *can* do instead of the things that you *want* to do. The whole idea was that doing things that you're able to do will eventually lead you to do things that you want.

I commented on the above post, telling the participant that if she continued to make these small, sustainable changes that in no time her diet would be where she wanted it to be. Because, really, that's the truth. Not just with diet changes but with anything.

If we keep doing things that we're able to stick to, things that we're able to say yes to, things that we feel so completely confident that we can accomplish, then sooner or later we're going to be doing things that we once weren't able to. Habits build, and consistent actions build.

So it got me thinking.

Is our fixation on the goal getting in the way of actually reaching it?

It's easy to want something that we don't currently do or have. That really is the nature of goal setting—to plan and strive for something that's currently out of reach. And goal setting is absolutely important and necessary for us to stay motivated and create plans for ourselves.

But if you get up one day and you really want to run a twenty-five-minute 5K but your legs are feeling sore, do you not run? Or do you run a slow 3K instead? Because that's what you can do that day.

A lot of people wouldn't run. Running a slow 3K wasn't their goal. Running a fast 5K was.

If you want to start consuming less sugar but you love having a Coke every day, do you give up on the idea entirely? Or do you cut out the sugar in your coffee instead? Because that's what you *can* do right now.

A lot of people would give up on the idea entirely.

Instead of focusing on the goal, focus on the right now.

Goal setting and big picture thinking don't mean anything if you don't decide what your next step is. And I mean the next, small, doable step.

And goal setting doesn't mean writing a gold star on a sticky note and slapping it on the fridge. It also doesn't mean announcing it to the world and hoping that because someone other than you heard, it's going to happen. Goal setting really should be called goal mapping. Because the only way to effectively get to a goal is to map out how you're going to get there.

This means breaking down the goal into tasks and to-dos, and then breaking those tasks and to-dos into smaller ones. Seems pretty straightforward. Yet we can still screw that up.

Why? Because our first step is too often too big.

BUILDING ANY GOAL-SETTING FOUNDATION WITH NONNEGOTIABLES

And now you're thinking, *Ok, so where do I start? How do I make sure that the things I'm focusing on are broken down enough so I won't give up?* This is where your nonnegotiables come in.

The other day I was speaking with a frustrated client and she said to me, "But Amy works out for one hour every day and she has two kids...why can't I do that?"

In my response I said to her "...because Amy has created non-negotiables for herself. This is one of them."

I want you to think of a few daily or weekly tasks that you do. These can be small tasks. Or they can be larger things that you complete on a regular or semi-regular basis. Getting up at 9:00 a.m., making eggs for breakfast, drinking two litres of water, taking the dog to the park, calling your mother, walking to work, getting to the gym, doing your skincare routine, going on a hike, or meeting with friends.

Now, can someone talk you out of doing any one of these things for a day? Can *you* talk yourself out of doing any one of these things? If so, it isn't a nonnegotiable. It is not high enough on your priority list to be completed regardless of what is going on in your life.

Creating nonnegotiables for yourself is one of the first steps in successful goal mapping.

I've always loved the analogy of health and travel because those two have so much in common, and it's such a great way for us to make sense of something with the help of something already so well known to us. The thing about goals is that if we just take an approach to them that is similar to what we do with travelling, we wouldn't find ourselves failing so often.

On January 1, you don't wake up in the morning deciding that you want to visit twenty-one countries in the year and then show up at the airport the same afternoon. Travel always comes with hiccups and delays. And to ensure that you don't give up and get on a flight back to your hometown, you either need a lot of grit and determination, or you need a well-planned itinerary. Or both.

And I won't downplay the need for a lot of grit when it comes to tackling goals, especially if we're setting long-term ones. But why put yourself through unnecessary hardship when you have many other things going on in your life that you need to worry about?

This is where nonnegotiables come into play and why they can be so helpful.

Think of your nonnegotiables as your foundation.

For example, "Not staying in a hostel" can be a nonnegotiable for travel. It also lays a foundation of what your accommodations will look like.

Let's dive into some details.

WHAT ARE NONNEGOTIABLES?

Nonnegotiables are regular activities or tasks that you have set in stone. No matter the situation, rain or shine, chaos at home, kids are screaming, boss is calling—you get them done. Because that's just the way it is. These are things that neither you nor anyone else can convince you not to do.

WHO NEEDS TO CREATE NONNEGOTIABLES?

Everybody. Literally, everyone. We should all have a small list of daily things that give us a sense of routine, pride, and accomplishment.

WHY DO WE NEED NONNEGOTIABLES?

At the end of the day, we all want to feel accomplished and productive. And we want to lay our head on the pillow knowing we did exactly what we set out to do for the day. Creating intention and a plan of action for each day drives success. Once we have nonnegotiables, we have a foundation. We have a list of things that we can rely on to give us that feeling, even when life gets absolutely out of hand.

The magic of nonnegotiables is that they fit seamlessly into your lifestyle and routine. To the point where you no longer have to consciously plan them in your schedule. They just get completed.

That's when you can create new, larger ones or build on your current ones.

For example—my current nonnegotiable is to walk seven to ten thousand steps a day. Soon I'll be at a point where my nonnegotiable will be to walk nine to ten thousand steps a day, eliminating the days where I'm below nine thousand.

HOW DO WE CREATE NONNEGOTIABLES?

Well, we start small. Smaller than we might think. Again, these should be able to fit into your current life and routine. They shouldn't disrupt any already important routines or commitments you have in your life. Rather they should enhance them.

Take a look at current things you do to enhance your health, nutrition, or fitness. Ideally, you want to start with something small that you do every day. It can be drinking two litres of water or getting seven hours of sleep. Maybe it's as small as doing a ten-minute journaling or meditation exercise a few times a week.

Regardless of what it is, remember that you cannot be talked out of it. You cannot be convinced to give it up for a day or week. It is now a part of who you are.

This is exactly how you, too, will get to a point where an hour of exercise a day is just who you are and what you do.

Later on in this section we're going to revisit nonnegotiables and how they play an important part in your goal setting and mapping process. For now, I want you to start thinking about what sort of nonnegotiables you can add into your daily routine.

GETTING STARTED ON GOAL SETTING

I want you to think about a time in the past when you had some large goals. Let's get excited about them! Maybe it's when you were little, and you wanted to become a ballerina. Maybe it's when you first decided that you wanted to become a mother. Perhaps it's when you decided you were going to go for a promotion at work.

For me, I can go as far back as being about thirteen years old, having the goal of being a veterinarian. Fast forward to about sixteen, and I wanted to go to the Olympics in swimming. Fast forward another eight years and I wanted to go to the CrossFit Regionals the year after I started training CrossFit!

If we take a step back and look at these goals individually, they're all pretty large and lofty. And if we're being honest, they're also a bit out of reach. Now, this is not to say that being a vet, getting to the Olympics, or competing in CrossFit are unrealistic achievements by any means.

But at the time they were for me.

At the time I was unaware of the idea of inclusive goal setting. I was setting these goals for myself based on an idea of them. Based on the reaction and feeling they gave me when I thought about them. Not based on what I could realistically achieve. I didn't give a thought about what they meant for me long-term. And I didn't think past the initial reaction.

Now, a reaction or strong emotion is enough to get you going. But unfortunately, it's not enough to sustain you.

When I was little, I had strong emotional attachments to animals. That, at the time, is all I knew. The feelings that animals gave me was all I needed to set a goal for myself of being a veterinarian.

When I was a competitive swimmer, there was this girl I would train with every day. I remember so vividly the coach saying she would make it to the Olympics. I had this feeling deep down in my gut that I, too, needed to make it to the Olympics. I just had to. Little did I know that the feeling I had in my gut was just my competitive jealousy getting the best of me. I didn't even really care about actually getting to the Olympics. Needless to say, I didn't.

When I started CrossFit, I started training with all of these women who were (and are) incredibly fit. And some of them were making their way to Regionals—a weekend-long competition held in a big city. This is step two in making it to the CrossFit Games. Again, my competitiveness kicked in and I set a goal for myself of wanting to go to Regionals.

I never pursued any of these goals. I barely even made a plan for any of them. They were 100 percent reactionary goals.

Let's take a look at the differences between inclusive and reactive goal setting.

INCLUSIVE	REACTIVE
Well thought out	Volatile
Repeatable	May not fit
Fail - Proof	Temporary
Customized	Uneducated

Figure 2

The truth about reactive goals is that they're volatile. They likely don't make sense in your lifestyle. They give you temporary positive feelings, but they're based on a fleeting moment, not who you are as a person. And most importantly, you create these types of goals without any knowledge of how to actually get there or how to achieve them.

Inclusive goal setting is the exact opposite. These types of goals are well thought-out. They're customized for you and your lifestyle. And done right, inclusive goal setting can actually be failproof. If you can successfully complete an inclusive goal-setting session once, that means you can complete it again and again, forever. Always setting and achieving goals.

When we do a goal-setting session successfully, we take into consideration all the areas of life. That means all the roles and responsibilities we, as busy women, have. Maybe you're a daughter, a mother, a girlfriend, a coworker, a pet parent, or a friend. These are all equally important things that need to play a role in your goal-setting process. And the roles that you play the most are the roles that will most affect the goals you set.

For example, let's say the majority of your time is spent as a small business owner. You wear many hats, and you play many roles. And because you're a high achiever and a go-getter, you decide that you want to also run a marathon. This is a personal goal that you know will make you happy. What is the most *valuable* thing for a business owner? Time. And what does training for a marathon take up? Lots of it. And so, was this an inclusive goal? Or was this a goal that was set based on feeling like you "should" be doing something?

Let's think of some other ways to set some inclusive goals for ourselves.

WHO MOTIVATES YOU?

Now, let's say you're having a hard time coming up with a goal that fits your lifestyle and *also* gets you excited. This, of course, can be a problem because we're so involved in many areas of our lives that we sometimes might feel we genuinely cannot set any new goals for ourselves. And trust me, I get it. But this is a problem because *you* don't get to go after what you want. And what you want matters.

Think about someone who gets you motivated. This person can be closely tied to you or they may know who you are. Who has a direct influence on you? How have they motivated you? And what has it provided you with?

Looking into areas of your life that spark excitement is important in this goal-setting process. Those areas likely are outside of your comfort zone, and likely are not taking up a lot of room on your plate. For example, I get so caught up in writing, running a business, coaching, and trying to be successful in my career that I think to myself, *There's no way I could put anything else on my plate!*

Then I look at my brother. He has multiple jobs, a family, and is one of the fittest men on the planet. After taking a moment to look at his life, I say to myself, *Actually, I can have more. I can do it all.*

I can then set myself a fitness-related goal that puts energy back into life so I can show up for my business as a better version of myself.

Later on in this book we'll talk more about surrounding yourself with people who allow you to level up and take on goals that will get you excited.

WHAT ARE YOUR COMMITMENTS?

The last area that you want to consider when setting goals is the commitments you have in your life.

Commitments and roles can be very closely tied, or they can be totally separated. Some of the roles you play as a busy woman might have you tied to certain commitments each day or week.

Using myself as an example, my role as a business owner has me committed to weekly meetings, content creation, writing, and coaching, amongst many others. There's a certain amount of hours each week that I must dedicate to the growth of my business.

As a fiancée, I must commit to the growth of my relationship by spending time and effort on date night, conversations and quality time, vacations, wedding planning, etc.

Laying out the commitments you have will help you understand how much time and effort you're already pouring into other things. This will allow you to visualize how much time and effort you have for something new.

Next, let's talk about how we can use these strategies in goal setting to create some real-life, super exciting yet totally achievable and realistic goals for yourself. Inclusive goals.

"If you want to be happy, set a goal that commands your thoughts, liberates your energy, and inspires your hopes."

— ANDREW CARNEGIE

SETTING YOUR GOALS

Goal setting can be challenging. But there are some things to remember every time you do a goal-setting session that will help you get crystal clear on where you want to go.

1. **Create positive goals:** Reframe negative goals into positive ones to keep you from approaching them with a negative attitude. For example: change "I want to stop eating so much junk food" to "I'd like to focus on nourishing my body better." With negative goals, the initial motivation often comes from, of course, a place of negativity. You might want to stop eating so much junk food because you feel unattractive or unconfident. These negative connotations can actually lead to negative self-talk, demotivation, and criticism along your journey. And who wants that?
2. **Brainstorm:** Don't just write the first thing that comes to mind. Take into consideration everything we just went through together and be inclusive when setting goals. Sit with it for a little while and make sure it not only speaks to you butalso fits in your life.
3. **Be optimistic but realistic:** If you set an unrealistic goal, it may discourage you early on from continuing your journey to achieve it.
4. **Evaluate your goals and reflect upon them:** Feedback is

critical. And self-generated feedback is more powerful than externally-generated feedback. After setting a goal, sit with it and assess or visualize how well you are going to do achieving it. Try setting up a schedule where you can check in on your progress regularly. Every day for short-term goals, maybe every month for longer-term ones. This is an opportunity not only to check in with yourself but also to see if there's a need to redefine your goal along the way. This is all a part of the process.

5. **Tell others about your goals:** When we share our goals, we're more inclined to exhibit accountability and strength in committing to them. If we tell a friend about a goal, and months later that same friend asks us how it's going, how are you going to feel if you have yet to take a step?

6. **Believe in your abilities:** But also know it's always okay to reevaluate your plan. And it's okay if things don't go according to plan. Remember that any progress toward a goal is a good thing.

"Goals affect the intensity of our actions and our emotions—the more difficult and valued a goal is, the more intense our efforts will be in order to attain it, and the more success we experience following achievement."[13]

"We are motivated by achievement and the anticipation of achievement. If we know a goal is challenging yet believe it is within our abilities to accomplish, we are more likely to be motivated to complete a task."[14]

It's time to write down some inclusive goals for yourself.

Goal 1: _____

Goal 2: _____

Goal 3: _____

SETTING YOUR CLEAR PATH

Congratulations. You now have three clear, inclusive goals for yourself. How do you feel!?

This part of the book is all about taking action. Executing. We know now that all the planning in the world means nothing without putting it all into action. Just like inclusive goal setting really means nothing unless we have a clear path forward.

Let's get to work.

I don't know how many times clients have come to me twelve days into trying to accomplish a goal and are overwhelmed with how difficult it turned out to be. So they give up. And it's so unfortunate because they didn't actually fail to achieve the goal, they just failed to properly map out how they were going to get there.

Goal mapping is an absolutely crucial part in any journey. Especially a health or weight loss journey for a busy woman like yourself. Because of how many things are going on all the time, setting a goal without a clear next step is like being trapped in a glass room with your destination on the other side. You can see it, you can sense it, but there are one hundred doors and each one you open has either a rushing river, a rocky mountain to climb, or a massive overgrown forest. Basically imagine any situation where every step you take, you're unsure whether it was the right one. You may step on a slippery rock and get rushed down the river. You may step on an unstable ledge and trip and fall. You may get lost in the forest. It's easy to use nature as an analogy here because often the vast landscape that nature has to offer can feel so overwhelming. And that's the same feeling you get when you set a goal for yourself without any clear steps.

Now imagine you open a door and the same landscape is there, but there's a staircase. There may be distractions, the stairs may get wet, dirty, or whatever. And so you proceed with intention and caution, but at least you proceed. Because you know, without a doubt that the step in front of you is the best path in getting to your goal, your vision.

When it comes to creating a path for your goal, the more you know about what it takes to get to your goal, the better. And so I usually ask myself three questions when I start mapping things out.

1. What do I currently know about what it takes to get to this goal?
2. What are topics I might want to research that are associated with my goal? OR What do I still need to learn about this goal?
3. Who can I use as a guide on my path to reach my goal? (We're going to dive deeper into building your life raft—the people that support you and keep you afloat along your journey— later in this book.)

To keep things simple, I'm going to use a personal goal I have of being the fittest I've ever been at thirty-five. So let's answer these three questions using that goal as an example.

WHAT DO I CURRENTLY KNOW ABOUT GETTING TO THIS GOAL?

I know I have to look back at when I was my fittest before.

I know I have to review previous training regimes and workouts.

I know I have to define "fit" and what that means to me in the context of this goal.

I know that I'll have to do some sort of combination of running, CrossFit, high intensity interval training (HIIT), swimming, and cycling.

I know that I'll likely have to hire some sort of coach for extra accountability.

WHAT DO I STILL NEED TO LEARN ABOUT GETTING TO THIS GOAL?

I have to research how my body will react to training in my thirties versus my twenties.

I know I'm much busier now, so I'll have to plan how I'm going to make this fit into my schedule sustainably.

I'll need to adjust my nutrition routine, maybe recalculate my macronutrients (more on this later in the book).

I'll need to work on my mindset and stress management, maybe take up meditation or yoga.

WHO CAN I USE AS A GUIDE IN REACHING MY GOAL?

A running coach.

A nutrition coach.

A friend or accountability partner.

A training buddy.

A family member.

Questions I like to ask myself when choosing someone who will help me achieve this goal are:

- How are they like me?
- Do they share the same or similar values as me?
- Have they gone through or are they going through a similar journey? Or have they helped others to a similar destination?
- How can they help?
- What do they offer? More importantly, does what they offer work for me in my learning and application style?

FINDING YOUR NEXT TO-DO

Once you've answered these questions, it's time to determine your very next step. If you've done any research or reading at all in the world of goal setting, you know what SMART goal setting is. SMART goals are:

- **S**pecific
- **M**easurable
- **A**ttainable
- **R**elevant
- **T**ime-based

But maybe you didn't know about smart**ER** goals, which:

- Evaluate
- Review

I'm all for smart goals and smart goal setting, but where I put these smart goals in the goal mapping process might be a little different. See, I'm all about the vision. As an entrepreneur, my biggest job is being a visionary. It's important for me to keep my creative, out-of-the-box thinking and as a result, set some creative and out-of-the-box goals. I'm a strong believer that the goals you set should get you fired up. They should get you excited! Because if they don't...well...why would you act on getting to them?

Breaking down your goal into specific, measurable, attainable, relevant, and time-based goals is the next step in creating some action items and actually getting your butt moving!

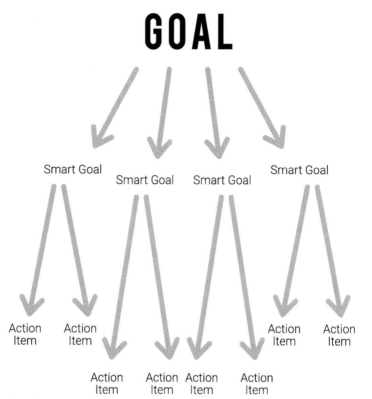

GOAL

Smart Goal Smart Goal Smart Goal Smart Goal

Action Item Action Item Action Item Action Item

Action Item Action Item Action Item Action Item

Figure 3

If we continue with the same goal of me being my fittest by thirty-five, the next step is breaking it down into some smart goals. Examples of smart goals:

- run a twenty-five-minute 5K
- reduce my sugar intake
- increase daily activity level and reduce sitting
- gain flexibility in my lower body to reduce aches and pains

Now we can pair these smart goals with some action items:

Goal—Run a twenty-five-minute 5K	**Action**—Schedule in two runs a week
Goal—Reduce sugar intake	**Action**—Schedule in one day a week to allow myself treats
Goal—Increase daily activity	**Action**—Walk for fifteen minutes before work
Goal—Increase flexibility	**Action**—Practise yoga twice a week

Here are some other examples of what action items could look like:

- walk 10,000 steps a day
- workout four to five times a week
- hire a coach
- eat two servings of veggies at lunch
- find an accountability partner

schedule workouts in my calendar like they're work meetings. The truth is, we never give up on something that we're 100 percent confident in doing. And that's exactly why we're doing these steps. We're going to be clear and deliberate with planning out our action items so that we can always feel the utmost confidence in our actions.

TAKING ACCOUNTABILITY FOR OUR ACTIONS

You have your next step; you know what you're going to do. Everything is set in place. Now it's time to hold yourself accountable and act. When you don't take accountability and things start to go awry because you don't feel ownership, you go into spectator mode and just watch as things fail. If you thought it would fail from the outset, it's even worse because you go into that, "I told you so" mentality, which nearly always becomes a self-fulfilling prophecy.

If things start to go wrong and you can step into solution mode, you can start to figure out what's going wrong and try and fix the problem. People who are successful are people who go into solution mode. Whether you find this accountability through yourself or through another person is up to you. But you have to tie yourself to your action items and take ownership. This is what will separate you from the pack.

Now, I want you to start picturing where this first step is going to lead you. This is your next opportunity to do some future journaling.

How do your days look? What are you doing? What are you not doing? How are you feeling?

I want you to visualize your journey over the next few days and months. You can even start to visualize the bad days that are ahead. I would be lying if I told you that all days on your route to your goal would be rainbows and butterflies. But if we can visualize and mentally prepare for tough days ahead of us, we can be sure we're going to have a much higher chance of pushing through.

I then want you to think about what happens if you do not stick to this first step. What if you aren't able to hold yourself account-able, or no one else is able to hold you accountable? What does that mean for your whole journey? What does that mean for you and your emotions? Do you give up on this first step and thus give up on the whole goal altogether? Or do you switch gears? Maybe think of an alternate route and push forward.

Enter the ER of SMARTER goal setting. Evaluate and review.

The reality is that there is always more than one path to a destination.

Having a plan B is never a bad thing. And plan B doesn't mean you need to change the destination. It just might mean you switch some steps on the path there. Because really, that's all you ever need in life—a plan and perseverance.

Section 3

BUILDING FROM THE GROUND UP

I live by the idea that the world is full of a million shades of grey. It's ignorant of us to feel like we need to subscribe to one way of thinking, especially with regard to something that is so personal, unique, and ever-changing as a diet or a health journey. And the reality of this book is that it's not teaching you some fancy new way of losing weight. This isn't glamorous. And I like it like that because I'm not about tricks, I'm about truth. And what makes dieting and weight loss so confusing is the fact that each diet has been a truth to someone. Each diet has worked for someone out there. Most of the time, temporarily.

Now, unfortunately where we start to get hurt and act on mis-information is when these people dive into a diet that gives them temporary success and start preaching it as the way of doing things. Most people who do this have zero foundation, no lifelong habits, and are seeing success based on unsustainable efforts. These are people who have decided to skip the actual hard work of creating sustainability and instead opted for temporary ab-checks.

I'm about to introduce to you the BODZii pyramid. And soon you'll see exactly how most people jump straight to the tip of the pyramid to gain quick results and neglect the most important part of sustainability—the foundation.

Now, it's important to note that this section of the book is all about giving you the facts on how to achieve sustainable results and what to focus on in your journey—and, most importantly, *when*. These are the straight-shooting, no bullshit, works-for-every-human-with-a-brain-heart-and-digestive-system facts.

What you do with these facts is up to you. It's important to me that you be as neutral as possible as you move forward reading this section of the book, because this is information. What you DO with the information is dependent on you as a unique, beautiful, wonderful, busy, human woman. We've spent the first part of this book talking about how to approach information and what to do with it. So you have the tools to sort through this section and figure out what applies to you and your goals and what may not.

Let's go.

THE BODZII PYRAMID

I founded BODZii in 2016 with the intention of arming women with the tools and confidence they need to see forever results. Since day one, sustainability has been my number one priority, and so everything that I teach and preach revolves around that. With that in mind, I created the BODZii pyramid. This pyramid really encompasses our philosophy and approach on coaching women in their weight loss journey and guides us on what to be focusing on, and when, along the way.

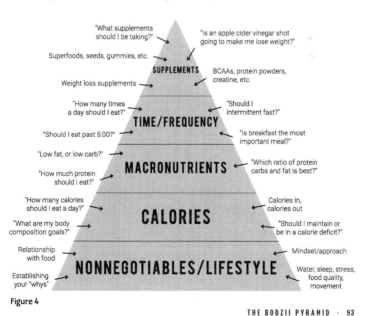

Figure 4

If you follow me on social media, you know that I have been talking about the foundation being the most important part of a successful journey for a long, long time. And you might also know that I have been a CrossFit coach for longer than I have been a weight loss coach. For about three years while coaching, I managed our basics, otherwise known as our foundations, program. Each new member coming into the gym needed to go through five classes with me to work through the nine foundational movements of CrossFit before attending their first group class or immersing themselves in the community. This was my opportunity to help them lay their foundation and really reinforce my belief that the length and strength of your success will be determined by how strong your foundation is.

The members graduating from the foundations or basics program were injury-free and they were moving correctly and more safely. They had a solid foundation they could build on.

In 2015, I had shoulder surgery that prevented me from working out at the level I wanted for about two years. Because I neglected to take time and build solid foundations, I was prone to injury. I thought I was saving time in getting to my goals by skipping some of these basic levels of training. I later made up for it by spending time in a sling instead.

I get it. You're at your wit's end from years of yo-yo dieting. You're frustrated and after all the years of putting in effort, you're still not where you want to be. And so of course you want to see results quickly. Maybe you've even seen amazing results in the past but weren't able to hold onto them, and so you're constantly being pulled in the quick, unsustainable direction again. Because your mind is going, "Well, I've done it before...maybe

I'll just do it again and figure out the rest later." Unfortunately, later never comes and you're left feeling stuck.

The faster you get results without prioritizing the basics, the quicker your results will disappear.

I get a lot of questions about weight loss. Like, a lot. And some of the most common questions that I get are along the lines of:

"Which supplements should I be taking?" "What are your thoughts on apple cider vinegar?"

"Should I eat after 5:00 p.m.?" "Should I be doing intermittent fasting?"

"How long should I be waiting between meals?"

And I give the same response every single time when I get a question like this: "How's your sleep, stress management, water intake, nutrient intake, protein intake, and activity level?"

I usually get a pretty stunned look after that and slowly the truth comes out.

"Well, I'm not great at getting to the gym. Definitely could be better at eating veggies. I sleep about four to five hours a night…"

> Every question you may have about supplements, timing, and frequency should not be answered until you have a rock-solid foundation and a good understanding of calorie balance and macronutrients, so we won't be discussing them in depth in this book.

The great thing is, you've already spent time learning about the importance of nonnegotiables, so now let's talk about the five nonnegotiables that we prescribe every single one of our members.

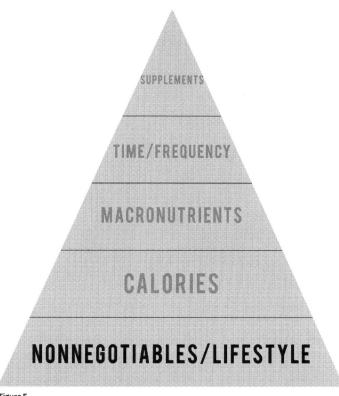

Figure 5

NONNEGOTIABLE #1: SLEEP

PRESCRIPTION: SLEEP SEVEN TO EIGHT HOURS EACH NIGHT

"By helping us keep the world in perspective, sleep gives us a chance to refocus on the essence of who we are. And in that place of connection, it is easier for the fears and concerns of the world to drop away."

—ARIANNA HUFFINGTON

The decision to go to bed early is the catalyst in making a day's worth of good decisions.

A NIGHT OF GOOD SLEEP LEADS TO REGULATED HORMONES

Let's go through the basics of our hunger hormones and particularly how they are affected when we don't get enough sleep.

There are three hormones to talk about here—ghrelin, leptin, and neuropeptide Y.

Ghrelin is a multifaceted gut hormone that's released by the stomach, the pancreas, and the brain. One of its main roles is to tell us that we're hungry. So it would make sense that ghrelin levels are at their highest right before a meal. We often call it the "hunger hormone" because it stimulates appetite, increases food intake, and promotes fat storage.

Leptin is essentially the opposite. This hormone is produced in the small intestine and works to regulate energy balance by inhibiting hunger. Leptin levels will be at their highest right after a meal. It does a great job of communicating to the brain when we have enough energy in the system, particularly in our fat cells, for the body to engage in an activity.

Neuropeptide Y (NPY) is a peptide that's found in the nervous system—the brain and the spinal cord. The NPY pathway stimulates an increase in appetite and food intake after exercise, energy loss, and fasts. Studies have shown that an increase in NPY is linked to cravings for carbohydrates as well.[15] There are other factors that can contribute to an increase in NPY levels, like insignificant protein intake.

These three hormones are best regulated when we get enough sleep.

And sleep deprivation can also affect your body's ability to regulate other hormones, such as the stress hormone called cortisol and the growth hormone which allows us to recover.

Getting enough sleep is crucial for maintaining healthy levels of our appetite-regulating hormones and our blood glucose levels.

A NIGHT OF GOOD SLEEP LEADS TO MANAGED EMOTIONS

You really don't need this book to tell you that when you're running low on sleep, you feel more irritable, testy, on edge, and maybe even just straight-up frustrated all day.

The interesting thing about the relationship between sleep and our emotional regulation is that there are some pretty significant things happening in our system that we need to be aware of.

My hope in cultivating simple knowledge surrounding our body and brain is so that we can (a) understand and have that "aha!" moment and (b) proceed to make better, well-educated, and conscious decisions.

Any sort of sleep deprivation—especially when chronic—can significantly impact your emotional well-being, outlook on life, relationships with others, and mental health.

Have you ever snapped at your partner for leaving a kitchen cupboard door open after you were up all night working? Impulsive and intensive emotional responses are much more likely after a poor night's sleep. Even a single night of sleep deprivation sets us up to react more strongly and impulsively to negative or unpleasant situations, according to research.[16] And as a lot of us do, we're working on many days of sleep debt. Just think about what that can do to our mental health.

Although there is much research to be done on this topic, there are some things we do know about our brain and how it changes after a poor sleep.

Research shows sleep deprivation increases activity in the rapid emotional response center of the brain—an area known as the amygdala.[17] This part of the brain controls many of our immediate emotional reactions. When short on sleep, the amygdala goes into overdrive, causing us to be more intensely reactive to situations.

At the same time the amygdala is fired up, lack of sleep also hampers the communication between the amygdala and another area of the brain involved in emotional regulation—the prefrontal cortex.[18] This part of the brain handles a lot of complex tasks, and one of them is to put the brakes on impulsiveness.

So now we have one fired up, ready to charge part of the brain, and another that's meant to calm it down completely unaware of what's happening. Talk about a recipe for disaster.

If you're feeling like the world is against you all the time, constantly worried about the future, or in constant battle with your partner, it might be time to take a look at how you can improve your sleep.

There's a way you can fix this, and there's definitely a brighter future ahead of you if you prioritize that restful slumber.

A NIGHT OF GOOD SLEEP LEADS TO A CLEAR HEAD

Managing emotions is one thing, but making good decisions is another. The ability to make sound, thought-out, and well-intended decisions throughout the day is what ultimately shapes us into who we are as a human. When sleep deprived, our judgement and ability to make these decisions are tampered.

The prefrontal cortex—the area of the brain that handles planning and complex decision-making and enables you to make complicated, nuanced judgement calls that balance risk and reward—is especially hard hit by sleep deprivation.

As we now know, when low on sleep, you're more likely to be impulsive in your decision-making. Impulsive decisions tend to favour immediate rewards, rather than the best outcomes over time. You're also more likely to engage in risky behaviour, according to research.[19]

There's also fascinating research indicating that sleep deprivation makes us more likely to cheat—again, that's thanks, researchers think, to the depletion of our ability to exert self-control in favour of doing the right, but often harder, thing.[20]

You see why this is so important and crucial to our health and wellness in the long run.

Sound judgement, solid planning, and thoughtful decision-making—these are the important cognitive skills that help us thrive, succeed at work and in relationships, create stable lives, and live out our values. Sleep deprivation makes these important, grown-up life skills more difficult.

With all that said, it's pretty easy to understand why we "don't feel like ourselves" after a week of late nights and early mornings. Because really, we aren't.

WITH REGULATED HORMONES, WE CAN STAY IN TUNE WITH OUR HUNGER CUES

Finally, we can start talking about weight loss, particularly how everything we just talked about is so crucial to our progress. Whether you have a goal of losing weight, building muscle mass, being healthier, or increasing performance, the amount you eat is always important.

Not being in tune with when you're truly hungry or full can cause you to overeat. I feel like this is a no-brainer. If your body is not working properly to send signals telling you when you're full, you're not going to stop eating—right?

Maybe I'm just speaking for myself.

In other situations, since we now know that ghrelin levels are increased when sleep deprived, we know that we will feel more hungry than usual. This might lead to more frequent meals or snacking throughout the day, and ultimately to an increase in calories.

Why this is so important is because when trying to lose weight or be at our healthiest, we want to learn how to eat our meals until 80 percent full. Eating slowly, staying mindful of how our body and stomach feel, and eating to 80 percent full are crucial for things like nutrient absorption and digestion.

If you're practicing this on a good night's sleep, your hormone levels will be able to work in your favour to let you know when you're satiated. Satiety is really what we're aiming for. We're not looking for a full stomach, and we're definitely not looking for a post-Thanksgiving dinner belly. Instead, after a meal you should be able to feel satisfied, energized, and ready to move on with your day. Not ready to take a nap.

WITH MANAGED EMOTIONS, WE CAN TAKE THE EMOTION OUT OF OUR FOOD CHOICES

One of the hardest things for people to do when they have a weight loss goal is to start looking at food as fuel. The reality is that food has so many emotional, spiritual, and religious ties to it, that it can be extremely difficult for us to see food as having one job—to energize us.

I think food is quite a magical thing that can bring families together, create a sense of community, give warmth to an occasion, and bring a smile to faces. And it's these things that also lead us to see food as being so emotionally charged.

Our fond memories of events and occasions surrounding food can misguide us into thinking that it should always give us the same feelings. This is why it's so difficult to separate food from emotion.

Now, slap a poor night's sleep and some irritability on top of that already difficult task, and we're headed down a slippery slope toward a heaping bowl of Doritos for breakfast.

Maybe you have some sort of weird emotional tie to Doritos, I don't know.

Since we now know that quality sleep can help manage our emotions, hopefully we can move forward prioritizing our sleep, and thus regulating our irrational food choices.

WITH A CLEAR HEAD, WE CAN MAKE A BETTER EFFORT TO WORK OUT OR MEAL PREP

There were a couple of important things noted above that I want to bring to your attention again—sound judgement, solid planning, and thoughtful decision-making. These three things are what will lead us to either work out or sit on the couch. To meal prep for a couple of days, or order takeout.

I believe I've said this before: if I could bottle consistency and sell it, I wouldn't have to work another day in my life.

Consistency is what drives results.

Planning drives consistency.

Decision-making drives planning.

If you have a goal of losing weight, you have to be in a consistent caloric deficit. There really is no other way around it. And to be in a consistent caloric deficit, we need to be able to plan out our meals and track our food to make sure we're staying within that deficit.

What it comes down to is the ability to make that decision. And really, that's what weight loss is all about. Making decisions throughout your day that are going to take you either a step closer or a step farther away from your goal.

So make the right decision—get a good night's sleep.

Now, the best way to get into good sleep patterns and to improve the quality of sleep is to make sure you develop good habits.

I've put together ten things that you can do to improve your sleep.

1. Lay Off the Caffeine

As any coffee lover knows, caffeine is a stimulant that can keep you awake. So avoid caffeine (found in coffee, tea, chocolate, cola, and some pain relievers) for four to six hours before bedtime.

2. Turn Your Bedroom into a Sleep-Inducing Environment

A quiet, dark, and cool environment is the best way to achieve peaceful sleep. To achieve such an environment, lower the volume of outside noise. You can use earplugs or even simply turn on something to create white noise, like a fan or a humidifier. Use heavy curtains, blackout shades, or an eye mask to block the light that's a powerful cue telling the brain it's time to wake up. Keep the temperature comfortably cool and the room well ventilated. The room temperature will vary from person to person, so it's difficult to recommend an exact temperature.

3. Create a Bedtime Routine

A bedtime routine can cue your body to get ready for sleep. Make the transition from wake time to sleep time easier with about an hour of relaxing activities. Your body will start to recognize the routine and slowly start to wind down. What you choose to do is up to you, but it should be calming.

4. Use Light to Your Advantage

Natural light keeps your internal clock on a healthy sleep-wake cycle. Let light into your house while you sip your first cup of coffee to get your day going. If you work in an office, get out on your lunch break, or try and take regular five- to ten-minute walks outside to keep you from hitting those midafternoon slumps.

5. Keep a Consistent Sleep Schedule

Going to bed and waking up at the same time each day sets the body's "internal clock" to expect sleep at a certain time night after night. Try to stick as closely as possible to your routine on weekends and holidays to avoid a Monday morning sleep hangover. Your body does get used to waking up early, as awful as it may seem for the first few mornings.

6. Nap Early If at All

Many people make naps a regular part of their day, and that's great! Especially if you have an early morning shift. However, for those who find falling asleep or staying asleep through the night problematic, afternoon napping may be one of the culprits. The sleep drive is a real thing. It's pretty self-explanatory—sleep drive is your drive to go to bed nearing the end of the day. This sleep drive decreases significantly if we nap in the afternoon. Try and keep naps shorter and before 4:00 p.m.

7. Lighten Up on Evening Meals

I'm not a huge believer that no eating after 7:00 p.m. is the way to go, but it might be a reason why you're not sleeping as well as you could be. Eating a large, heavy meal thirty minutes before bedtime might be a recipe for insomnia.

8. Balance Fluid Intake

This can be tricky for a lot of people. Balancing your fluid intake can take some time of closely monitoring how your body responds and reacts to amounts of liquid. Drink enough fluid at night to keep from waking up thirsty—but not so much and so close to bedtime that you will be awakened by the need for a trip to the bathroom. Try drinking about a cup of water before bed and see how it makes you feel.

9. Try Exercising Earlier

Exercise can absolutely help you fall asleep at night. Exerting high levels of energy during the day demands that you get enough rest and relaxation in order for your muscles to repair themselves. However, exercising too close to bedtime might be the reason why you're not sleeping too well. Exercise stimulates the body to secrete the stress hormone cortisol, which helps activate the alerting mechanism in the brain. This is fine, unless you're trying to fall asleep. Try to finish exercising at least three hours before bed or work out earlier in the day.

10. Follow Through and Stay Consistent

It's always about consistency over perfection. Some of these tips you will be able to stick to more easily than others. Choose one to tackle at a time and make your changes small and manageable.

If you stick with them, your chances of achieving restful sleep will improve. That said, not all sleep problems are so easily treated and could signify the presence of a sleep disorder such as apnea, restless leg syndrome, narcolepsy, or another clinical sleep problem. If your sleep difficulties don't improve through good sleep hygiene, you may want to consult your physician or a sleep specialist.

NONNEGOTIABLE #2: MANAGE YOUR STRESS

PRESCRIPTION: PRACTISE STRESS LOWERING AND MINDFULNESS ACTIVITIES DAILY

Stress is the body's reaction to any change that requires an adjustment or response. The body reacts to these changes either physically, mentally, or emotionally. Stress is a normal part of life. The human body is designed to experience stress and react to it. Stress can be positive, helping us stay alert, motivated, and ready for danger. Stress can also be negative when we face continued challenges without relief or relaxation. A stressful event can be something physical, such as running a marathon; psychological, like worrying about an upcoming work deadline; or persistent, like chronic anxiety.

Here are four of my favourite best practices to help relieve yourself of stress:

1. Meditation

Meditation has become more and more popular over the years with apps like Headspace, Calm, The Meditation App, etc. I remember when there was a stigma around meditation for our mental health—like we didn't really need it, or that we could just eliminate stress on our own if we wanted to. As stress and mental health awareness have become more talked about, meditation seems to have a bigger place in people's lives. Meditation can come in all different forms, and it's important to find out what way works best for you. Refer back to section one of this book for great meditation and mindfulness practices.

2. Exercise Variance

BODZii as a company works closely with the world of Cross-Fit—a high-intensity, very successful, and incredibly effective form of exercise. Also a very stressful form of exercise. As we now all know, there are many forms of stress, including good and bad. A good level of stress is what we are exposed to in the gym. Stresses on the body that trigger positive hormonal change for muscle development can include high impact and weight/load exercises.

What we also know is that there is such a thing as too much of a good thing. Constant, high intensity in the gym might be a reason why you're feeling overly stressed out. Exercise of course is a fantastic way to relieve stress, and walking into a gym with blasting music and a heavy barbell to throw around sounds like a good way to blow off some steam. Balancing out your exercise with something a little lower intensity is also a good way to manage stress. Try going for a thirty-minute to hour jog—or even longer if you love running! Take a new route and extend your usual run by twenty to thirty minutes. Take a yoga class and experience a different kind of intensity through mindful breathing and body awareness.

Not only will you feel relaxed after your time spent slowing down, but your body will also thank you for it the next time you hit the weights as well!

3. Nature

There are a number of ways in which natural environments may promote human health by reducing stress. Natural environments can often provide the setting for physical activity, with numerous studies reporting the beneficial effects of "green" exercise. Exercise in outdoor settings has been reported to be more restorative and stress-reducing than indoor exercise. Walking in green spaces and other outdoor settings has been linked to increases in self-esteem and overall mood levels. Reported intentions to continue participation in walking exercises was higher in participants using the outdoors when compared to those in indoor settings.

So what does this mean? Get outside! Plan a monthly activity for you and your friends to do outside. Hiking, swimming, snowshoeing, skiing, or biking. Or even take your daily workout routine outside once in a while and go hike some stairs. Find yourself a park and some friends and set up some interval stations for you to go through together.

4. Eliminate Sugar

Although sugar might not have a proven direct impact on anxiety or stress levels, it does appear to worsen anxiety symptoms and impairs the body's ability to cope with stress.

If you're someone who suffers from panic attacks, mild or severe, you might benefit from eliminating sugar from your diet. Sugar causes tiredness, a lack of mental alertness, and sometimes even blurry vision. These can come across as anxiety-like symptoms, causing anxious people to have a heightened awareness of their anxiety throughout the day.

Try supplementing sugar out with alternatives like stevia, applesauce, honey, and/or maple syrup. Make sure to watch your daily intake and limit yourself to under eight grams of sugar (natural included) a day!

If you're a sweet coffee lover, head to Starbucks and ask for a pump of sugar free syrup in your coffee for some sweetness.

NONNEGOTIABLE #3: MOVEMENT
PRESCRIPTION: WALK SEVEN TO TEN THOUSAND STEPS DAILY

We know moving is important. A study published in the *British Journal of Sports Medicine* found that those who adhered to a walking program showed significant improvements in blood pressure, slowing of resting heart rate, reduction of body fat and body weight, reduced cholesterol, and improved depression scores, with better quality of life and increased measures of endurance.[21]

But it's not only your physical body that will benefit from walking.

The act of walking is also a proven mood booster. One study

found that just twelve minutes of walking resulted in an increase in joviality, vigour, attentiveness, and self-confidence versus the same time spent sitting.[22] Walking in nature specifically was found to reduce ruminating over negative experiences, which increases activity in the brain associated with negative emotions and raises the risk of depression.[23]

Getting seven to ten thousand steps in a day can seem overwhelming, especially if you have a desk job. But little movement snacks add up—yes, movement snacks. Little moments throughout the day that you dedicate to five to ten minutes of movement.

Start your day with a walk: If you can get 2,500 steps before you head to work in the morning, you're putting a big dent in that 7,000 target.

Park further away: Heading to an appointment or going grocery shopping? Park in the farthest parking spot and walk.

Ditch the Uber: Save money and gain some steps instead.

NONNEGOTIABLE #4: STAY HYDRATED
PRESCRIPTION: DRINK 2.2–3 LITRES OF WATER DAILY

For active and busy women, hydration is so incredibly important. The effects of even slight dehydration can have a huge impact on your daily performance and mental clarity and alertness throughout the day.

If you're of the 70 percent of North Americans who could potentially be suffering from chronic dehydration, this next part is for you.[24] It's time to make some educated decisions on how you structure your day, with the goal of staying well hydrated. Here are five ways to help:

1. Combat Dehydration with Nutrient-Dense Foods

Of course, water is the first thing that comes to mind when thinking about hydration. But sometimes that's not the best or the only answer. Those who simply don't like the taste of water can use different fruits and/or veggies to give a more palatable taste to the liquid.

To stay hydrated, you also need more than just water. Electrolytes and carbohydrates are crucial to make sure the water you drink is being retained and put to good use.

While both nutrients can help your body absorb whatever fluids you drink, electrolytes—sodium, chloride, potassium, magnesium, and calcium—are especially important because they are critical to healthy nerve and muscle function. And all of these electrolytes can be lost through sweat.

2. Eat Your Water, Eat More Veggies

Outside of drinking fluids, you can increase your hydration by eating more vegetables. Vegetables (and fruits) are primarily made up of water. If you're not a fan of drinking water, eating more vegetables is an excellent way to keep your hydration levels up. Cucumber and lettuce contain 96 percent water, while zucchini, radish, and celery are close behind at 95 percent water.

3. Go Slow

Many people make the mistake of increasing their fluid intake too quickly. Rather than doubling your current fluid intake, start by slowly increasing by one to two cups per day. This incremental increase will help your body to gradually get accustomed to the new water levels. If you increase your fluid intake too fast, it will cause you to urinate more often, which actually makes you get rid of the additional water and some electrolytes.

4. Reduce and Reuse

Another tip to help stay on top of your hydration is to get a reusable water bottle to carry with you everywhere you go. Customize it, sticker it, write your name on it, or write motivational hydration quotes on it! Just stay away from plastic water bottles that are made with bisphenol A (also known as BPA, a chemical that seeps into foods and drinks and may lead to negative health effects). Instead, use a glass or carry your own stainless steel water bottle. Bonus—you'll be keeping plastic out of your recycling bin! Stay hydrated, save the planet!

5. Drink Herbal Teas

If you are in the mood for something warm to drink, herbal teas are another great form of hydration. Herbal teas feature therapeutic benefits that may help with inflammation, stress, digestion, and headaches. Because herbal teas don't have any caffeine, they can be counted toward your daily water intake. Some examples of herbal teas are ginger, peppermint, and chamomile. If it's the middle of the summer, drop some ice cubes in and treat yourself to a delicious, iced tea!

NONNEGOTIABLE #5: PRIORITIZE FOOD QUALITY

PRESCRIPTION: ADD NUTRIENT-DENSE FOODS AND PROTEIN AT
EVERY MEAL

The reason why we don't promote one way of eating over the other at BODZii is because everyone has their own unique goals, unique body composition, and unique needs. Why would we all then eat the same foods? This may not lead to the same outcomes. Before making food changes, it's important to ask yourself what your goals are. From there, let's establish what foods would be best to include in your diet in order to see changes.

Nutrient-Dense and Nonnutrient-Dense Foods

Nutrient-dense foods are those rich in micronutrients such as iron, potassium, magnesium, calcium, and omega-3s. Fruits and vegetables are usually the first things that come to mind. Nonnutrient-dense foods are foods that are low in nutritional value. Things like cookies, ice cream, French fries, etc., would be considered nonnutrient dense.

Calorically Dense versus Noncalorically Dense Foods

There is a common misconception that calorically dense foods are "bad," although foods like avocado and salmon are high calorie. Fruit tends to be higher in calories but also rich in nutrients. Things like green vegetables are ideal for those who are trying to maintain a calorie deficit since they are not only nutrient-dense, but also noncalorically dense.

Combining these two categories together will help you understand which foods will be more beneficial to your health and your goals. If you're in a caloric deficit and feel like you're hungry more than not, eating nutrient-dense and noncalorically dense foods will be ideal. If you have more calories than you know what to do with, you can choose more calorically dense foods that might be a little less nutrient dense in order to fulfill these needs.

Ok, but why is protein so important?

Here's why...

- A high protein intake boosts metabolism, reduces appetite, and changes weight-regulating hormones.[25]
- Replacing some carbs and fats with protein increases levels of satiety (appetite-reducing) hormones, while reducing your levels of the hunger hormone. This significantly decreases hunger and is the main reason protein helps you lose weight. It will help you consume fewer calories throughout the day overall.[26]
- After you eat, some calories are used for the purpose of digesting and metabolizing the food. This is called the thermic effect of food (TEF). Protein has a much higher thermic effect (20-30 percent) compared to carbs (5-10 percent) and fat (0-3 percent).[27]
- Due to the high thermic effect, a high protein diet allows you to burn slightly more calories throughout the day through natural digestive processes.[28]
- Protein makes you burn more calories around the clock, including during sleep.[29]
- Protein can have a positive effect on cravings and eliminate wanting to reach for those late-night snacks.[30]
- At the end of the day (our very busy day), losing weight is not the most important factor; it is keeping it off in the long-term that really counts. Many people can lose weight, but

most end up gaining the weight back, and a higher protein diet can also help prevent weight regain.[31]

- Eating plenty of protein can help prevent muscle loss when you lose weight. It can also help keep your metabolic rate high, especially when combined with heavy strength training.[32]

Nonnegotiables are meant to build a foundation that you can fall back on. This is what will ultimately keep you consistent and progressing as a busy woman. Executed properly, these nonnegotiables should become a part of your day-to-day life. They should become a part of who you are as a woman who prioritizes her health and happiness. However, that does not mean they will always become second nature or easy. They might. But they also might not.

And I say this because I don't know how many times clients have come to me saying, "Ugh, Robyn, I just wish getting my steps in was easy. I feel like I'm always planning when I can get a walk in."

Yes, of course. Because you're busy.

Getting seven thousand steps in a day isn't just going to magically start happening on its own after a few weeks of effort. It's always going to be an effort, but you're always going to make it a priority. That's what sets you apart, my dear.

UNDERSTANDING CALORIES

Continuing to climb up the BODZii pyramid, we next approach calories.

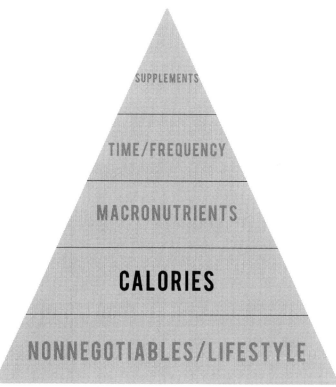

Figure 6

So what is there to know about calories? Balancing your calorie intake can be overwhelming. There is so much information out there on how much we need to eat to lose weight. Of course, I'm here to educate you first, and then take you through a way to determine your own specific needs. You might be able to breeze through this next section if you're already well-versed on basic nutritional science and information. But as you probably know already, a refresher on the basics is always a good thing.

What is a calorie?

Calories are units of energy. Our bodies need calories for everyday functions like breathing and keeping our hearts beating. Active bodies require more calories in order to keep up with energy demands.

We get calories from food, which come from four different sources. These sources are called macronutrients. These are carbohydrates, fats, proteins, and alcohol. Each one of them gives us different amounts of calories.

Carbs and proteins provide four calories per gram, fat provides nine calories per gram, and alcohol provides seven calories per gram. All except alcohol are considered essential, which means we need to be consuming these regularly for optimal health.

How much food we eat is always important. However, calorie counting is not the be-all and end-all. As previously mentioned, there are many different factors to consider when looking at nutrition, and knowing how much energy (a.k.a. calories) we need in order to reach our goals is only one of many avenues to consider when reaching for optimal health and wellness.

WHAT IS ENERGY BALANCE?

Energy balance is the difference between your energy input—or the number of calories that you put into your body—and your energy output, or the number of calories you burn each day.

Simply put, the equation is:

$$\text{energy balance} = \text{calories in} - \text{calories out}$$

As I mentioned at the beginning of this section, there's so much information out there on what we need to do in order to lose weight. The hard part is finding what works for you. The one thing we know will work for you (and everyone else) is being in a calorie deficit. We know this to be true. And honestly, that's partially what makes this one of the most frustrating things in the world.

How can weight loss, one of the most *frustrating*, complicated, nuanced, annoying, rollercoaster, emotional journeys, be broken down into such a small, simple equation?

And why does it seem like that equation never adds up to what you want!?

Honestly, this is exactly why there's only such a small section of this book dedicated to talking about a calorie deficit. Because the important work is not about what causes weight loss, it's about how we achieve it. How do we achieve this calorie deficit, and more importantly, how can we stay in it long enough in order to see the results we want?

In order to just get you started, I'm going to give you two ways to figure out your calorie deficit.

This first way is a super simple, three-step route.

1. CALCULATE YOUR CALORIES

Take your goal body weight and multiply it by twelve. If your goal body weight is 150, multiply it by twelve. 150 × 12 = 1800. Your daily calorie goal is 1800 calories.

> Goal body weight in this case is a weight that you see yourself at your leanest. This is not the actual goal body weight that will achieve happiness and balance. For some, they may be the same number. But for most, they will not be.

2. CALCULATE YOUR PROTEIN FOR THE DAY

Keep in mind that you get protein from all sorts of foods you eat throughout the day. The amount of protein you need can be met by a variety of sources, including eggs, oats, nuts, broccoli, lean meat, peanut butter, cheese, chickpeas, and more.

Take your goal body weight and multiply it by one. If your goal body weight is 150, you need 150 grams (g) of protein.[33]

3. START TRACKING YOUR FOOD

Use MyFitnessPal and hit that goal, in this example 1800 calories and 150 g of protein. Do this consistently for four weeks and see what happens!

The second route is a bit more complex and takes the amount of activity into consideration. If you're exercising regularly and need more of a customized approach to accommodate your workouts, choose option two.

First, we need to know how to calculate our calories out. Your calories burned will depend on a couple of things.

- your basal metabolic rate (BMR)
- your daily energy expenditure

Your BMR + your daily energy expenditure = your total daily energy expenditure (TDEE).

SO HOW TO CALCULATE OUR TDEE?

The first and easiest way to do so is here: www.tdeecalculator.net.

It is an amazing resource that not only calculates your TDEE but will also give you a breakdown of macros based on your caloric needs.

The second way is to take your body weight in pounds and multiply it based on the suggestions below:

10–12: Sedentary: little to no exercise, desk job

12–14: Light Active: exercise three to four times a week for thirty to sixty minutes

14–16: Active: exercise four to six times a week for thirty to sixty minutes

16–18: Very Active: exercise four to six times a week for one to two hours

19–23: Elite: exercise five to seven times a week for two to four hours/double sessions

Now that you have your TDEE, you have your maintenance calories! This is the amount you need to eat on a regular basis to maintain your current body weight.

FINDING YOUR CALORIES IN

In order to do this, you will need to track your food intake. At the end of your day of tracking, you'll end up with a total number of calories consumed. This can be compared to your estimated total amount of calories needed. The results can look like any one of these possibilities:

Perfect Balance

If you end up with a zero at the end of your energy equation, you've found a perfect energy balance. In this state, you won't gain or lose weight. Perfect energy balance is for people who are in the maintenance stage.

Positive Energy Balance

If you end up with a negative or RED number, it means you've eaten over your allotted calories. You've achieved the right balance for weight gain. For some people, like pregnant women, growing children, and weightlifters who are trying to bulk up, this is a healthy state. If you want to focus on building muscle mass, this is also a great option. For best results in a muscle building phase, maintain a positive balance of 200-500 calories daily.

Negative Energy Balance:

If you end up with a positive or GREEN number, you've found the energy imbalance necessary for weight loss. This imbalance is also called an energy deficit. It means that you've tipped the scales to slim down. For best results you want a negative energy balance of roughly 200–500 calories per day to lose 0.5–1.5 pounds per week.

Just to note, the colour of the number or the words "positive" or "negative" mean nothing beyond the equation. They are just numbers that will help you choose which path to take. And depending on which tracking app you're using, the colour of the numbers may change. I used MyFitnessPal.

HOW TO CHANGE YOUR ENERGY BALANCE TO LOSE WEIGHT

There are only three ways to change your energy balance. In short, you have to either reduce your caloric intake, increase your energy output, or combine the two options to achieve the calorie deficit needed for weight loss. The right method for you depends on your health history, your lifestyle, and your personal preferences.

1. REDUCE YOUR CALORIE INTAKE

If you can't exercise or if you absolutely hate to exercise, you can reduce your caloric intake by 500 per day to lose weight. Once the weight is gone, however, people who choose this option usually have a hard time keeping the weight off. Sustainability of weight loss increases significantly when paired with exercise. So if you hate to exercise, maybe it's time to build that growth mindset and approach it with a different attitude...right!?

As you slim down, your metabolism and body composition change. That means that your energy output number will decrease, thus you'll have to keep decreasing your energy input even more to reach the desired energy balance. In short, you have to eat less. For many people, eating less is not reasonable or sustainable for the long-term.

2. INCREASE YOUR PHYSICAL ACTIVITY

You can also change your energy balance by exercising more. But burning an extra 500 calories every day with a workout can be difficult for some. You would need to be able to do this every day in order to achieve the desired result.

3. COMBINE INCREASED ACTIVITY AND DIET CHANGES

Making small adjustments to both your caloric intake and your physical activity is generally recommended as the most reasonable and sustainable method of weight loss.

Using this method, you can burn a few hundred extra calories with a workout and cut back calories by eliminating dessert or high-calorie snacks to reach your goal. It is also the best way to maintain your weight after you've slimmed down.

Understand that this method can take a little bit for your body to adapt to. Putting your body in a caloric deficit for the first time could come as a shock to your body, so it might take some time to see changes. Stick to it for a few weeks and adjust your calories to reflect your activity level as needed.

If you're deciding on which route to take when it comes to weight loss (cutting), weight maintenance, or weight gain (bulking), here are a few things to take into consideration:

- The majority of your time should be spent in maintenance. Maintenance calories are where your body experiences the least amount of stress. Any body change, even positive change, is registered as stress to the body and a constant calorie deficit or surplus isn't sustainable. If you've recently done a cut or gain, maybe it's time to get back into energy balance and give your body a break. Generally speaking, any woman who has been eating under 1500 calories for more than a few months should start eating at their maintenance again. Slowly increase calories and monitor your weight—if you are increasing caloric intake and maintaining your weight, great! This means you're reverse dieting your way back to your maintenance calories.

- Every cut you go through should only last eight to sixteen weeks, depending on where you are at in your life and how your body responds to calorie deficits. Because a cut should only last this long, your accuracy, precision, and discipline with tracking your food needs to be on point to make sure you're in the negative energy balance. This level of precision can become taxing, not just to your body, but to your mind as well.

- Each weight gain phase you go through should be taken with the same approach—to only last roughly eight to sixteen weeks. Being in a constant surplus of calories will eventually lead you to put on unwanted fat, when really we just want to focus on muscle building for a shorter period of time.

Now that you have a better understanding of how to approach calories, let's talk about what calories are made up of: macronutrients.

MACRONUTRIENTS

Next up on the pyramid is macronutrients.

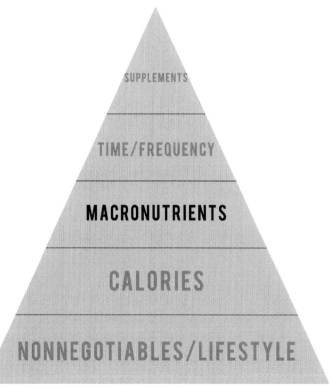

Figure 7

If you were to eat purely based on calories, you would be completely ignoring the fact that your body uses different macronutrients for different purposes. Bodybuilders have known for years that you need to pay attention to your macros, and the effectiveness of this system has caused it to transition from being a tool of athletes, to becoming a powerful nutrition tool for all.

Counting macros means paying attention to the ratio of each macronutrient you consume throughout the day, allowing you to adhere to diets like keto, which require roughly 70 percent of your food to be from fats and as low as 5 percent from carbs.

It also allows you to treat your diet like a science lab. You can tweak your ratios to discover where you feel best, etc.

So let's talk about macronutrients. As mentioned in the last section, our calories consist of macronutrients which are necessary to our survival. Carbohydrates, fats, and proteins are the three essential macronutrients.

CARBOHYDRATES

Carbohydrates are our main energy source. Our bodies rely on carbohydrates for ready, easy-to-use energy. We can find carbohydrates in the form of starches, sugars, and fibre. Our bodies break starches and sugar sources down into simple sugars, which our bodies use or store as energy.

Our bodies are unable to break down fibre, which then passes through our system and keeps our digestive system moving.

Healthy starch sources come from whole grains like quinoa,

whole wheat pasta, rice, starchy vegetables like sweet potatoes and squash, and legumes.

Natural sugar sources come from dairy like milk and yogurt, as well as fruit.

Although natural sugars are found in products like maple syrup and honey, the body breaks these sugar sources down very quickly, similar to what it does with table sugar. Because of this, we recommend sticking with dairy or fruit if you want natural sugars, as they contain additional beneficial properties like protein, fibre, and micronutrients that other sugar sources do not have.

Other carbohydrates to avoid are the types that have been processed in a way that have stripped that food of beneficial nutrients (such as white flour and fruit juices) or have added sugar like flavoured yogurts, granola bars, and jams.

Sweeteners are an alternative when trying to control your carbohydrate content and sweet tooth. Safe sweeteners for use include stevia and sucralose.

FATS

Fats have many roles in the body. Major functions include being a source of energy (we can store endless energy away as fat), absorption of vitamins A, D, E, and K, satiety, healthy brain function, reducing inflammation, and much more.

When it comes to fat there are three sources: unsaturated, saturated, and trans fats. We recommend avoiding trans fats at all costs. These are primarily man-made fats that are found in processed foods. Luckily, Canada banned artificial trans fats from our food supply in 2018.

Saturated fats are found in animal products and many processed/packaged products. Saturated fats are often solid at room temperature (such as marbling on meat, butter, and cheese).

Unsaturated fats are the fats we recommend you choose most often. These are found in plant and vegetables sources like vegetable oils, nuts, seeds, and avocado, as well as fatty fish like salmon. Although many red meat products are sources of saturated fat, they are still okay to have in moderate amounts, no more than two to three times per week.

Avoiding high fat dairy products is recommended. Aim for cheeses with around 20percent milk fat, and around 2percent milk fat for milks and yogurts.

PROTEIN

Proteins are part of every cell in your body. They are needed to build and repair muscle, skin, nails, hair, and other tissues in the body. They are also needed to build hormones and enzymes in the body.

Recommended protein sources include chicken, turkey, fish, lean red meat, tofu, and cottage cheese. Protein sources that have a mixture of carbs and fats include legumes like lentils and chickpeas, nuts, seeds, and eggs. And, well, we've already covered why protein is so important.

Now, what do you do with this information? You start to track your intake of each one.

WHERE DO YOU START?

At this point, you should have an idea of how many calories you currently eat and how many calories you need in order to get to your goal (weight loss, maintenance, or weight gain). But how do you determine what ratio your macros should be?

This is where you can experiment. Treat your body like a laboratory and dedicate some time figuring out how your body feels its best.

Here are a couple things to know when figuring out your macro ratios/splits.

1. START WITH PROTEIN

As an active person, you will need about 0.8–1 g of protein for every pound you weigh. (If you weigh over 150 pounds, getting more than 150 g of protein may not be sustainable for you as a busy woman. Take your goal body weight discussed in the calorie section of the book and use that as your target.) That means a 150-pound female will need 120–150 g of protein per day.

If that 150-pound female decides to eat 150 g of protein a day, that equals 600 calories (150 g × 4 calories/gram) each day of her allotted, let's say, 2000 calories.

That's equivalent to 30 percent of her total daily calories. Now we know she has 70 percent left to split between carbs and fat.

2. SPLIT UP CARBS AND FATS

If this same female's goal is to maintain her body weight but work on losing fat and building muscle at the same time, she might want a nice balanced split of carbs and fats, dedicating 40 percent to carbs and 30 percent to fat.

Her macros would then be 150 g protein, 60 g fat, and 200 g carbs.

(Thirty percent of 2000 calories is 600, and 40 percent of 2000 calories is 800. Each of these are then divided by their macro's calorie per gram, which is nine for fats and four for carbs).

3. CHOOSE YOUR PATH

If her goal is to lose body fat, she is going to want to maintain all the muscle she has in her body. Going through a weight loss phase needs to be monitored so that she does not lose skeletal muscle mass at the same time.

We know that protein helps build and maintain muscle mass. After she reduces her caloric intake, let's say to 1800, she can keep her protein higher at 30 percent, maybe even 35 percent, and then adjust her fats and carbs to reflect how her body feels.

If her goal is weight gain, we can reduce protein slightly and start to use carbs to our advantage by fueling our muscles and giving us lots of energy for weight training and potentially heavier lifting! If you're on a weight gain phase, pairing it with weight training is the best way to see success. Maybe her split now will be 25 percent protein, 50 percent carbs, and 25 percent fat.

4. EXPERIMENT

When in doubt, try something, track it for at least thirty days, and record your results. If energy is low, aim for additional carbs. If you are having a hard time with muscle mass, increase protein. If you are leaning out too quickly and your performance, mental clarity, and daily energy levels are low, increase fats.

5. PRIORITIZE ENERGY

Remember that the most important thing before even thinking about macronutrients is making sure that you are eating enough. If you're feeling tired or you're not making progress, it might not be your macros. It might just be that you need to eat more to support your level of physical activity, or that you're still eating a little too much for how active you are.

With a lot going on in your life, your job is to keep your journey as simple as possible. As mentioned early on in this section, no meal timing or supplementation is going to matter if you don't have the basics down. And that's really what this book is all about—empowering you to focus on seeing the growth and results you want through mastering the basics.

Now that this chapter is coming to a close, I feel it's necessary to remind you that every bit of information in this section is just that—information. And as we know, information is not power. It's what you do with this information that will determine your success. If that means you decide to start tracking your food to better understand how your body responds to a certain intake, wonderful. If that means that all you're going to focus on is your nonnegotiables because your goal is to live a healthy, balanced life with no body composition goals in mind—also wonderful! Your goals are yours. They make you, you.

Section 4

TRUSTING THE PROCESS

We've built our mindset, we've worked on goal setting, and we've gathered the necessary information, but it's still easy to get really impatient. So in this section, let's talk about how we can practice our patience by tracking our progress and collecting information.

We praise people for being money conscious, tracking their spending and setting monthly budgets, yet we tend to judge people for doing the same with their nutrition and fitness.

Why?

The healthiest way you can approach a health and weight loss journey is with curiosity and patience. Too often we get caught up in the need to know all the answers right away. We need results yesterday, and we need the number on the scale to go down right now. And if I asked you *how* you would like to lose weight, you'd likely say something like, "I don't care! Just get me there."

We've lost all sense of curiosity when it comes to how our body works, how it responds to food and exercise, and what it really needs to thrive. We care about how we look in a mirror, how our clothes fit, and how we are perceived by others. It's sad.

Carol Dweck (remember her?), author of *Mindset: The New Psychology of Success*, comments on studies of curiosity and age in simple, binary terms. Children are greatly affected by their caregivers in terms of putting the child into either a growth or fixed mindset. Dweck described the language that tends to encourage a growth mindset, phrases such as "let's find out," "I wonder," and "what if...?"[34]

Curiosity and a growth mindset clearly go hand in hand. As you know by now, we're all about harnessing that growth mindset in order to see a truly successful health journey. A part of that means putting yourself in that "let's find out" state of mind. If you can understand your body and its unique physiology, you'll have forever control on how to make yourself feel good, increase muscle, decrease body fat, and increase energy.

Imagine, for a moment, that level of control.

You want to lose fifteen pounds of fat while maintaining energy? You know how to do that.

You want to increase muscle mass and feel strong? You know exactly how to get there.

You want to maintain your body weight and focus on regulating your hormones and stress levels? You got this.

The truth is, you can have all of this. And as you go through life and your goals change, you can know exactly what you need to do to get there. The catch? You need to be curious. And you need to be patient.

Approaching a journey with curiosity means you're not approaching it with frustration. You're not approaching it from a place of lack. You're approaching it with an open mind, an eager mind, a curious mind. You're interested in what works for your beautiful, unique body. You are focused on you, not anyone else. You treat your body like a laboratory. You take trial and error as getting you one step closer to your goal, not as a waste of time. Approaching your weight loss journey with curiosity is like creating your own personal Google database where you get to answer all the questions you've ever had about weight loss with answers specifically made for you.

How cool is that?

With this new-found curiosity comes a need for patience. You won't find your perfect answer right away. And as mentioned, you may have to go through some trial and error. All of this takes time. But it's worth it if you can maintain curiosity and that growth mindset.

I know you know this already. And I know as you're reading this, you're likely shaking your head saying, "Yes, Robyn, we've covered this already." But our intentions for how we want things to go can easily get derailed by the emotions of the moment. And after years of yo-yoing and not seeing the results you want, the next fad diet that pops up on social media can be very shiny and attractive.

Earlier in this book we talked a lot about establishing a solid "why" before starting a journey or setting any goals. Having solid motivating factors can make being patient a whole lot easier.

A big part of trusting the process is seeing progress. The truth is it's a whole lot easier for us to stay motivated and feel we're on the right path if we can actually see ourselves moving forward. And this is exactly why I'm such a huge condoner of collecting as much data as possible along our journey. The more information we have, the more progress we can see.

THE IMPORTANCE OF OBJECTIVE DATA IN YOUR HEALTH AND WEIGHT LOSS JOURNEY

Self-love and body-positivity culture have been some of the best things that could have ever happened to the world of dieting. No longer are men and women tied to a single goal, and no longer is eating healthy and working out tied to just one thing—the number on the scale.

We're starting to embrace the multitude of ways we can measure our personal progress.

To get a full 360 degree look at someone's progress, however, we need to take a look at both the subjective and the objective data. And this, I believe, is the best way to keep someone motivated, learning, and moving forward.

SO WHAT IS OBJECTIVE DATA?

Objective findings come through either measurement or direct observation. Objective data cannot be argued—it is measured and observed through vitals, tests, and physical exams.

What are examples of objective data or measurements when it comes to personal health, fitness, and nutrition?

- body fat percentage
- body fat mass
- skeletal muscle mass
- waist, hip, and chest measurements
- weight
- average running speed
- weight lifted

Some of these, of course, are a lot easier to retrieve than others. And since some objective data can be simpler to retrieve, we tend to put more weight on it. Pardon the pun.

And although it shouldn't *always* weigh more, there are times when this type of information blazes the trail in guiding us forward.

WHY IS OBJECTIVE DATA SO POWERFUL?

The road to sustainable weight loss and lifelong health is a long one. It's indeed lifelong. And a very winding one at that. Often, you'll have to identify not only what your next steps are, but what sort of shoes you need to be wearing to make them.

In other words, you need to set goals. And you need to figure out how to get there. That's always step one.

Step two is attaching metrics to those goals to make sure you're actually moving in the right direction. Think of it as a compass reading or a GPS. Your GPS reading is showing you real-time data on each step you're taking, letting you know if you're moving toward your destination or farther away.

The most powerful and important word there is "real time." When it comes to weight loss or body recomposition, there's no obstacle greater than time. The reality is that if we don't see results fast enough, we lose interest and/or motivation. We just talked about patience. Gathering information like weight and body measurements can give us that real-time information. We can collect this type of information periodically with the intent of being able to visualize our progress.

The second most powerful and important word is "showing." As just mentioned, setting out a system where we can visualize our progress gives us some instant gratification—again circling back to the power of real time. Because if we cannot see progress when we look in the mirror, at least we can see it on paper.

Let's talk about weight for a moment because it has to be one of the touchiest subjects of them all. But it really can be such a powerful tool in guiding us to our goals—of course, if approached with the right attitude and mindset. And this is exactly my reasoning for spending so much time focusing on exactly that—mindset. When it comes to something like weight, because of its volatility, it can make someone's day, but it can also break someone's entire journey. And if you happen to weigh yourself on the "wrong" day—after a big meal, maybe when you're on your period, or when you're stressed out after a big work meeting—you'll see a number on the scale that you don't want to see, and your whole journey will be thrown off because of those three numbers.

Like...what? Why?

Because you didn't weigh yourself frequently enough.

Hear me out.

Figure 8 shows us five data points. With just five points, it's hard for us to get a grasp of what is really happening. We see a spike from point 1 to 2. And we see a bit of a drop between points 2 and 5 but it starts to level out. Overall, there's not a whole lot we can take away.

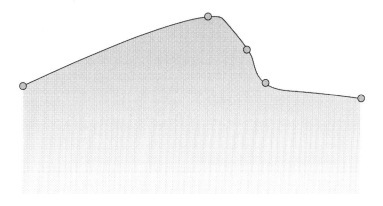

Figure 8

Figure 9 is better at showing us a little bit of a trend. But we can definitely get thrown off or distracted by the spikes. This client was great at weighing herself multiple times a week. But imagine she didn't, and she only happened to weigh herself on the days when weight was up (see circled data points in Figure 10). She would believe she's not making nearly as much progress as she actually is.

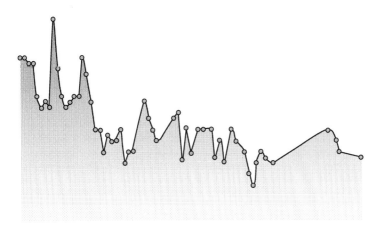

Figure 9

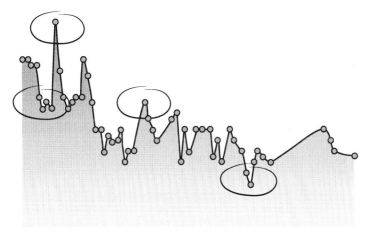

Figure 10

Or let's say she weighed herself only on a day where she had hit a new low and then a week later she collected data again, and it was a spike. She'd be missing all the information on what actually happened in between those two data points.

Figure 11 is much better at showing us a trend. Yes, we can see spikes, but more importantly, we can see that every spike is always lower than the previous spike, and every low is always lower than the previous low.

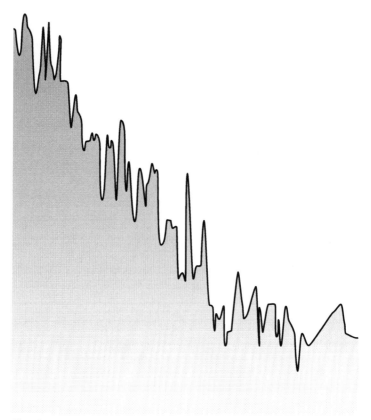

Figure 11

Figure 12 is three full months of collecting data three to five days a week. And there's no denying that there was a significant amount of weight loss.

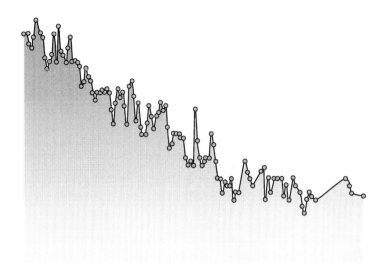

Figure 12

When on a weight loss journey (or a cut), weigh yourself every day. By doing this you'll take the "weight" off of each individual number, and you'll put the importance and focus back on the overall trend.

Of course, everything comes with its downfalls. And collecting objective data definitely has its own.

In order to be an effective coach, it's important for us to understand that with power comes a lot of emotion. And we cannot belittle someone's intense, oftentimes negative emotion and its connection to the number on a scale. Even if we wish that this wasn't the case.

How can we be so happy with the number on the scale going down but then expect to be totally in check with our emotions when the number on the scale goes up? With every intense emotion, there is an equally intense, opposite emotion.

A coach's job is not to take the power away from the scale by deeming it a useless or unimportant tool, but instead to lead clients to understand *when* it's important. And so, understanding when to put weight on a certain metric is really what this comes down to.

It all comes back to mindset and how we approach things. Why move forward in life allowing something like an object (the scale) or a number (your weight) to negatively affect your progress when you can see it as an opportunity to build your growth mindset and use that same object and number to your advantage?

With a growth mindset, we believe we are limitless. We can always change our thought behaviours and patterns to help us move forward to align our actions with our goals.

OBSTACLE VERSUS OPPORTUNITY

OBSTACLE	OPPORTUNITY
Feeling hungry	Understanding hunger signals
All-or-nothing mindset	Learn how to do everything in moderation
Self-sabotage	Practising self-love and grace
Lack of motivation	Finding something that excites us and that we care about
Cravings	Practising discipline
Feeling unfit and anxious about going to the gym	Building confidence and strength
Not feeling worthy	Practising positive self-talk and self-worth
Bad relationship with food	Learning how to view food as fuel and understanding how to practise balance
Bad relationship with the scale	Practising collecting objecting data to help take the power away from a number
Holidays and birthday parties	Balance, control

Figure 13

Speaking of emotions, the journey to our goals is full of them. It's easy to get caught up in the emotion of having a really productive week, just as it's easy to get down on the feeling of being in a rut or hitting a plateau. Personal progress is never linear, and we can always expect to have days or weeks that make us want to give up.

On a really crap day, it's nice to take a look at how far we've come.

Because on those days you'll be able to look back and see that, over all the data you've collected in your journey, not all of it was moving you forward. Maybe the weight on the scale was up one day, maybe your hours of sleep for the week were dropping, or maybe your body fat percentage had stalled. Overall, however, you can see a trend in the right direction.

WHEN IS THIS IMPORTANT?

It will be more common to rely on objective data as we start our path to a new goal or start a long road to a healthier us. The further we get into our journey, the less we will have to rely on numbers to help us move forward. We'll be able to then rely on intuition to maintain results and also keep pushing the needle forward. (More on intuitive eating in a moment.)

Why? Because one of the ultimate goals is to not have to worry about motivation dropping, or the possibility of you giving up. The goal is to have the experience, the knowledge, and the passion to keep on that forward trajectory—even if it's just a small shuffle—without relying on a number. However, that takes time.

Of course, objective data will always hold an important place in areas like competitive sport where we rely on numbers to see where we stand against the competition. Working with someone who has a very targeted goal is an example of a perfect opportunity to use objective data as your primary way of measuring.

Someone who might be new to the world of health and fitness will benefit from measuring their progress in the form of strength progression, weight on the scale, or speed on and length of a run. Or a busy woman like you who has a ton on her mind will be able to rely on the data to keep her on track amidst her hectic life. Just to name a few examples.

After a certain amount of time, that same person will no longer feel the need to move forward on paper but will rather just trust that she is.

This is exactly how we can learn to eat intuitively. Yes, we need to relearn intuition. Relearn because of course we're born with it but lose it over the years of parents imposing their food beliefs on us, being surrounded in the schoolyard and cafeteria with friends and their lunch boxes, and then exposed to the world of Bernstein, Jenny Craig, Weight Watchers, mixed with massive restaurant food portions, the accessibility of food juxtaposed with the fear that we'll run out and then...well...social media. That son of bitch really f*cked us up. Sorry. I told myself I wouldn't swear in this book, but I felt like if there was one moment to do it, it would be directed at social media.

We unfortunately have been brainwashed into believing that there is one way of doing things. Or that we need to look a certain way. And social media has convinced us that anecdotes are truth. Sally on Instagram sharing a photo of her losing thirty pounds doing keto doesn't mean that keto is the way to lose thirty pounds. And Trish sharing the fitspo photos of her working out two hours a day doesn't mean that we all need to be working out that much if we want to lose weight. What we see on social media is not truth.

Now the thing about objective data is...well...it's your truth.

Now, as mentioned a couple of times, we know that a weight loss journey is incredibly emotional. And what's the opposite of emotion? Objective data! We can't ignore the many emotional ties food has, especially when it comes to events like birthdays, holidays, and weddings. We love using food to bring us together and to create connections. Now, unfortunately, the emotion can sometimes carry us away and cause us to lose sight of balance and what makes us actually feel good. Enter objective data.

I want to talk about an objection that I get all the time when discussing weight loss with women, and how using objective data can help us put something overwhelming into very clear perspective. The conversation is always hilarious to me because they can talk for an hour straight about their goals, what they want, how badly they want it, and how much and how long they've tried leading up to this moment in order to get it. Then one sentence can make the entire conversation absolutely null.

"But the holidays are coming up...so I'm not going to do anything yet. I'll wait until January."

Excuse me while I slam my head into the wall.

There are two things I want to talk about here. One, why this excuse is so detrimental to your growth; and two, why saying this strips away the one thing that actually works—consistency.

So let's break down the holiday season, shall we? If you're in Canada, you have Thanksgiving that really kicks things off early. Because as soon as the leaves start to fall and the turkey hits the plate, we get into holiday mode. And for us north of the border, this happens right at the beginning of October.

Then we have Halloween, which I really see as just a day to give yourself a sugar rush and plummet into a sugar hangover laced with anxiety.

Then we have American Thanksgiving, then Christmas!

Before reading on, you should know that Thanksgiving and Christmas are the top two on my holiday list. So it's important to note that this is being written by someone who easily gets caught up in the holiday season. I'm with you, girl. But if we break the season down into days—and include Halloween—we have three days. Seventy-two hours. That's three days we can indulge, drink, toast, go for seconds and thirds, and not feel remotely guilty about it.

Now, of course what about the office holiday parties, family gatherings, and friendly dinners? Sure, let's double it. That's six of ninety-one days; 6.5 percent of your holiday season that you can dedicate guilt-free to taking time away from focusing on your nutrition. The rest of the time, you build your hedge.

Building your hedge increases the distance between where you are now and falling off the wagon. The more time you spend building your hedge, the bigger, wider, and stronger that hedge gets, and the less effect your guilt-free days will have on your long-term success. Of course, we need to talk about the one thing that you need in order to build your hedge—consistency.

Not only are we building hedges, but we're building consistency in order to build that hedge. And building consistency takes time.

If you're looking to get results and you've tried so long to get them, then you should have no problem dedicating time to creating something you know will last. "Waiting until January" eats into that time.

The next time you have the chance to talk to someone about your goals, end the conversation with a commitment: a commitment to your current self and a commitment to your future self. And then act. Because now you know you have two things you can start doing as you continue through any holiday season. Stop making excuses and start building your hedge by looking at the holidays (a bit) more objectively and realize that you have a huge opportunity to create balance. And build your hedge.

Holidays are a perfect example of an opportunity to find balance between emotion and objective data. I want you to celebrate, of course I do. And I will always want you to create memories with family and friends. But I also want you to get results, and I want you to feel in control every step of the way.

WHAT OBJECTIVE DATA TO TRACK BASED ON YOUR GOALS

If your goal is to lose weight, you want to be tracking your food daily. With a weight loss goal, your objective is to be in a slight caloric deficit daily, and with that comes the need to track both intake and outcome. Your intake, of course, being the food that you eat.

Use an app like MyFitnessPal, Lose It!, or Cronometer to track what you eat. And if you're reading this and have a little voice in your head going, "Ugh, I hate tracking food, it takes so much time and effort," I have two things to ask you:

1. This is the way to find out your own personal truth. Isn't that what you want?
2. Is your attitude toward tracking preventing you from receiving the information you need to see sustainable results? Do you need to work on your mindset?

Your outcome is your weight. So weigh yourself daily to start collecting the information needed to see your trends.

Now, those two things are what you need to track to see weight loss. But as you know, we're about sustainable weight loss. So here are some other things you need to start tracking to build your foundation.

Sleep, steps, weekly workouts, and water intake.

Want to take it a step further? Get regular blood work to measure hormones like cortisol, T3, and T4 to make sure there's nothing else getting in the way of seeing the progress you deserve.

If your goal is to maintain your weight, and maybe go through some body recomposition, the best things to measure your progress are things like:

- food intake
- progress photos
- the way your clothes fit

It's unnecessary to track your weight (although it may be a good idea every couple of days just to make sure you actually are maintaining), and you don't need to be as precise and diligent with tracking your food every single day. Maintenance comes from continuing to track the basics that build our foundation: sleep, stress, workouts, water intake, and food quality.

By now, you should hopefully have a new, more constructive outlook on the numbers along a weight loss journey. You should be able to move forward in control, having taken back the power that the scale and calorie counting have held over you for so long. This, my dear, is where you thrive. Because numbers don't phase you anymore—they push you forward.

> "I came into this program being afraid of the scale. I took it way too seriously and I allowed it to really affect my emotions about my journey. It's weird how much I don't care about the number on the scale each day anymore, and how much I can focus on what's actually happening in the big picture."
>
> —MOLLO MILLER, A BODZII CLIENT

Section 5

BUILD YOUR LIFE RAFT

"You are the average of the 5 people you spend the most time with."

—JIM ROHN

The first time I heard this quote I was sitting in a room full of some of the best coaches, multiple six-figure and seven-figure business owners, and my mentors. I looked around and I was like, okay, I'm supposed to be here.

My mentor and business coach, Zander Fryer, quoted Jim Rohn while speaking to us about how we can level up in our business by attending events where we'd be surrounded by multi-million-dollar business owners. I believe, to my core, that Jim Rohn is right.

However, I would like to add that we do also have our own consciousness. And so maybe a better way to look at it would be that we are the sum of the five people around us, plus ourselves. However, the underlying intent of his quote remains relevant. Who you spend time with influences who you become. Your actions, thoughts, and especially your beliefs.

LEVELLING UP

In university, I was very unhealthy. I carried a lot of extra weight, I drank a lot, and I barely attended classes. Honestly, I believed that I was supposed to find a normal nine-to-five job and make 40–50K per year, and that was that. At the time, I also had next to no financial literacy, no real responsibilities or understanding of life post high school. My drive was low, my ambition was low, and I thought that life would sort itself out without me needing to do much. Now maybe that sounds like a typical seventeen-year-old. But when I look back, I remember that I grew up in one of the richest neighbourhoods in Eastern Canada. Before you get any ideas, no, I wasn't rich. I was *surrounded* by the rich. I was surrounded by kids who also had zero real drive, ambition, or dreams because they *actually* had their life already sorted out for them, whether taking over the family business, or relying on a trust fund to kick start their adult lives. I visit my hometown to see my family, of course, and I get asked quite often if I stay in touch with any of my friends from high school. The answer is no—I levelled up.

When I moved to Toronto and found art is when I really started to find drive, passion, and ambition. I *loved* creating. I actually liked working long hours to get assignments done. I loved being the creator and owning something that was bigger than me—a piece of art. I used to feel lazy, but creating art made me realize that I wasn't lazy, I had just been uninspired. I spent five years surrounded by artists who were better than me, trying to make something out of themselves. And let me tell you this—there is no one who works harder at creating a living for themselves doing what they love than artists.

But there was a gap. The gap was my health.

With the art world comes late nights, parties, alcohol, and drugs. It's unfortunate, but it's the truth. And I found myself slipping. I was raised on the belief that exercise and good sleep can cure anything. A bad day, a broken heart, anxiety, overwhelm, laziness—get a good sleep and get to the gym. That was my cure. My cure was slipping away, and I had to take a good look at my surroundings and who was present.

The CrossFit gym that I was working out at occasionally started to become a more frequent part of my life, to the point that I was there almost daily. And once I graduated art school, I was presented with a choice that I think really was the start of my current life: become a CrossFit coach or pursue a life as an artist. I said early on in this book that I don't have the greatest memory but, girl, do I remember this moment. I was walking home from the gym after having been offered the job and I was standing at a streetlight when I called my brother for advice. My brother was a CrossFit coach and owned a gym, and looking back, just the fact that I called him shows that I had already made my decision. I just wanted someone to acknowledge that I was making the right one, and I knew I would get that from him.

The next week I started shadowing classes and filled the gap that was missing in my life. I was now surrounded by people and an environment that would allow me to prioritize my health and fitness every single day. I levelled up.

Over the next three years I would become the fittest I have ever been. I was competing in CrossFit, maintaining 12–15 percent body fat, running half marathons, and squatting over 200 pounds regularly. I was beyond thrilled that I found a way to push myself and my body to these capabilities. As someone who was incredibly unfit and borderline unhealthy, I didn't think this was possible for me. But I immersed myself completely in the environment to make it happen.

But there was a gap. The gap was the sense of ownership and creativity that art gave me. Sure, I was proud of my body and my fitness levels. But remember that creating something bigger than me is what truly kept me inspired.

Owning a business—that was my next pursuit. Creating something that would marry my love of health and fitness with my passion for creation. That's what I wanted to do. And the thought of creating a website really fired me up at the time, so I went for it. Seven years later, I'm constantly surrounded by business owners and coaches who are making a true impact in the world, making a living doing what they love, prioritizing their health and mindset, and loving life.

I levelled up.

Now, as I grew older, I realized that I didn't need to be so dramatic and completely sever ties with anyone who wasn't exactly in line with where I wanted to go. My seventeen-year-old self didn't really understand that, but my thirty-one-year-old self realizes that maintaining friendships is just as important as editing your surroundings. Simply monitoring your contact with the people who may not be in line with you is all you need to do, unless you find them to be seriously dragging you down or even moving you backward. The truth is, if you involve yourself in a relationship that doesn't serve you, you're not serving the other person either because you're not allowing yourself to be the best version of you, which is ultimately a disservice to the people around you.

Imagine if I had not taken action in editing my surroundings back when I was seventeen. Imagine if I had not listened to what my gut was telling me, what my lack of passion was telling me, and what my surroundings were telling me. I've never really been one for reminiscing (maybe that's why my memory is so crap), so I honestly can't even tell you what that life would be like. But I can tell you it doesn't look like where I am now.

Lately I find myself wanting to be surrounded by mothers. My mother, my sister-in-law, and some of my best friends who are also moms. And I'm confident that when the time comes, I'll be the best mother I can be because I've surrounded myself with the people who will help me become that version of myself.

THE TRAITS OF A SUCCESSFUL YOU

I've always been a huge believer of ruthlessly editing your life. That means taking a look around you and seeing what is contributing to your movement forward and what's holding you back.

What are the qualities of the person (or people) you aspire to be like? Or maybe more specifically, what are the qualities of the fit, healthy, happy, and balanced woman you want to be?

And when you get to be her, what are the qualities of the fitter, healthier, happier, and more balanced woman you want to be then?

I can definitely help you out here because, well, we sort of have already gone through them all. And as we near the end of this book, maybe it's a good idea to summarize each of the five things discussed and translate them into traits that you can acquire as a human woman on a journey to sustainable weight loss and ultimately better health, more confidence, and increased balance.

TRAIT #1

She has an open, growing mind. The woman who is happier, healthier, more confident, and in better shape than you knows that she also isn't the happiest, the healthiest, or the most successful she can be. But that doesn't scare her. It fuels her fire. She believes she is limitless and that there's nothing she can't do if she sets her mind to it. The number one trait of a woman who will achieve sustainable weight loss is a woman with a growth mindset.

She will do weekly (if not daily) mindset work in the form of journaling, reading, listening, or watching. She knows that a journey worth pursuing isn't full of rainbows and butterflies. But that's not what she wants either. She knows that pride and accomplishment come from overcoming adversity. And she knows that in order for her results to stick, she needs to feel proud. She needs to have skin in the game. And eventually she will crave hardship knowing it makes her stronger, and it makes her better.

TRAIT #2

She executes. The woman who is happier, healthier, more confident, and in better shape than you knows that knowledge isn't power—implemented knowledge is. She knows how to filter the information that enters her brain, knowing that the more information, not the better. Because she knows that too much conflicting information is overwhelming and will actually prevent her from acting and executing.

She knows that something is better than nothing. And something imperfect is always 100 percent better than failing to execute a perfect plan. She believes in taking messy action. She also knows that just because something worked for someone else, it may not work for her. Because she knows she lives a unique life with a unique schedule, planning in accordance with what she wants and needs on all fronts of her life is important.

TRAIT #3

She focuses on what's important. The woman who is happier, healthier, more confident, and in better shape than you knows what to zero in on, and when. She knows how to focus on the basics and work her way up, knowing that her foundation will carry her through. She sleeps seven to eight hours a night, she manages her stress levels, she drinks 2.5–3 L of water a day, she gets seven to ten thousand steps in daily, and she prioritizes high-nutrient-dense foods. And when she wants to level up, she tracks her food, she collects the data, and she stays consistent.

TRAIT #4

She's patient. The woman who's happier, healthier, more confident, and in better shape than you knows that there's no rush. She knows that sustainability comes from learning the most about her body, and that means collecting data. She lives by "all data, no drama" while going through a cut and understands that collecting objective data is a guiding light in her journey and an absolute necessity in her growth. She knows that trends are more important than individual numbers, and that her worth is not tied to a size of pants or a number on the scale.

TRAIT #5

She's surrounded by others who are happier, healthier, more confident, and in better shape than she is. She seeks out people who will support her and influence her. She constantly is editing her social group to find people who are in line with her ultimate goals.

FINDING YOUR PEOPLE

Take a minute to grab a pen and a piece of paper. Or if you're like me and your hand can't keep up with your thoughts, grab a laptop. Let's do an exercise. Answer the following questions:

1. What type of person do you want to be? This can be health and weight loss related. It also doesn't have to be. Imagine you at your best self; who is she? Write down a few qualities or traits that she has.
2. Who are five people that you currently spend the most time with? What top three qualities do each of them represent?
3. Do they match who you want to be in the future? Do their

qualities match yours? Do they detract from or contribute to the person you are trying to become?

4. Who are five people that possess the qualities you desire? These people could be famous, celebrities, friends, family, relatives, on social media, the president...anyone! Lady Gaga, Beyoncé, Audrey Hepburn, Oprah, or your wicked awesome neighbour. Align this person with what you want. If you want to become a writer, list someone who is a *New York Times* bestselling author. If you want to lose 100 pounds, list someone who's already achieved that same goal.

5. How can you increase contact with them? Maybe you can't speak face to face with Oprah, unfortunately. Or maybe you can! If you're reading this book and are able to speak face to face with Oprah...please call me.

Here are three different ways you can increase your "contact" with these five people:

1. **Direct contact:** If you listed your neighbour as one of your top five people, go knock on their door this evening and ask if they want to go grab a glass of wine. If they're in your network but are maybe a few degrees of separation away, start asking others how you can get in contact with this person. This can be through email, phone, text, Zoom, whatever!

2. **Work products:** Have they written a book? Do they host a podcast? How can you immerse yourself in the life of this person through the content they have put out into the world? Perhaps they have a blog or a YouTube channel. Listening to this person speak or reading what they write can be just as powerful as speaking to them face to face because their content will do a really good job of conveying their consciousness.

3. **Visualization:** This is powerful stuff. It might seem a little woo-woo to you if you've never practised visualization techniques before, but they are a real thing. Ask any Olympic athlete and I guarantee you that they visualize their event before executing it. One of the most classic ways we can manifest the actions or consciousness of the person is by asking "what would X do?" in a situation.

Now, what will happen as you increase your contact with these five people in any of these three forms? If the difference in your consciousness levels is high, you are probably going to start off feeling like you just don't belong. They will probably talk in lingo and topics that are different from what you are used to. Even when they talk about topics you are familiar with, their perspectives can be totally different and not something you have looked at before. I often feel like this when I'm scrolling through social media or listening to podcasts of people I look up to. I catch myself saying things like, "What the heck am I doing here? I don't belong." But we have to nip that in the bud.

If you connect with them every day, even if for just fifteen minutes at a time, it's just a matter of time before your consciousness shifts to the new level. Eventually you will start resonating with the people you aspire to be. You will find that you start thinking on the same wavelength and start talking about the same topics as them. This thinking will then affect your actions, which will manifest into the results you see in life.

I get a lot of women coming into our program who have jobs or commitments that make it very difficult for them to achieve all the things they *think* they want and need. And I highlight the word "think" because I want to remind you that the point of this book is to get you to the absolute best version of yourself. And in order to do that, you always need to take into consideration the very things that make you, you. That includes being a mom. Even if you can't always get seven to eight hours of sleep every night—at least you try. That also includes being a shift worker who loves their job but might not be able to meal prep as much as they would like—but at least you do your best.

If you have things in your life that you are seeing as obstacles, before going and changing them all, ask yourself, "Is this an obstacle I need to eliminate? Or is it one that makes me, me?"

Since the pandemic, BODZii has been a 100 percent online community. And the beauty of that is we get to connect with busy women all over the world who are on the same journey to better health and sustainable weight loss. That means we've created a worldwide life raft for each member who joins our community. I know how hard it is to make changes in your personal life, let alone have those changes affect the people around you. One of my main focuses while building up this program is making it easy for women entering to feel like they belong and they have that unconditional support from their peers. Even if they feel like they may not have it in their own lives at home, they can find it through the BODZii program.

CONCLUSION

Your Next Steps

Every single time I listen to a podcast, have a call with my mentor, or attend a webinar or conference, the only thing I'm really asking myself throughout is, "What can I take away from this?" It's important to me that you end this book with a list of actionable items. A to-do list. Gosh, I love to-do lists. If you need me to rewrite all of Section 2 again and talk about planning and executing, I can... But the beauty of this is that you can just go back and reread it. It's there to remind you that nothing in your brain matters if you don't act on it. So let's get moving.

Here are some things you should have created yourself:

1. A WEEKLY MINDSET CALENDAR

Whether you have your calendar on your phone or in a physical agenda, slot in your mindset work as if it's a meeting with your boss. This is a priority, so make it one. Remember that mindset work doesn't have to take up a ton of time. It's the intention that matters.

2. A LIST OF DAILY NONNEGOTIABLES

There are five things that you are now working toward every single day:

1. walking seven to ten thousand steps
2. getting seven to eight hours of sleep in (when possible)
3. stress management (mindset work, journaling, taking a breath)
4. drinking 2.5–3 L of water
5. Getting protein and nutrient-dense foods at every meal

On top of these five, you can work to create your own personal nonnegotiables that will customize your journey and lay your own personal foundation. Maybe you like to do five minutes of stretching before bed each night. Perhaps you take a cold shower each morning. Or maybe you're already hitting the gym multiple times a week. Whatever it is, write it down.

Action item: take a photo of your nonnegotiable list and tag @ hustlebuthealthy on Instagram! I can't wait to see it and hold you accountable!

3. ONE TO THREE SMART GOALS AND ACTION ITEMS

Use the template below to list your goal at the top, SMART goals below, and action items you can take today to get started.

Action item: snap a photo of your template and share it with me on social media, tagging @hustlebuthealthy.

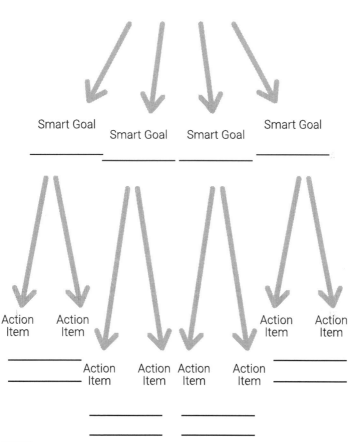

GOAL

Smart Goal　Smart Goal　Smart Goal　Smart Goal

Action Item　Action Item　Action Item　Action Item　Action Item　Action Item　Action Item　Action Item

Figure 14

4. YOUR PERSONAL CALORIE AND MACRONUTRIENT PROFILE

If you've read this book and are ready to take yourself through a calorie deficit, great! You should have all the tools you need for success.

5. A LIST OF PEOPLE (OR AT LEAST THEIR TRAITS) YOU WANT TO START SURROUNDING YOURSELF WITH

Make a list of your top five people and/or traits below:

....

....

....

....

....

As this book comes to an end, please remind yourself to come back to it whenever you feel you need to. I'm always here, waiting to give you the support you need, a virtual hug, or a smack on the butt if you will. And remember, nothing is sustainable if you don't become it first. So set off and become that woman that you know you deserve to be. It's time to prioritize you. It's time to set goals and achieve them. It's time for you to ask more of yourself and level up to a better, happier, healthier, more confident, vibrant, and energetic version of yourself. Because you know you're worth it, and I know you're worth it.

NOTES

1   Headspace (@@Headspace), "Meditation isn't about becoming a different person, a new person, or even a better person. It's about training in awareness and getting a healthy sense of perspective," Twitter, March 20, 2019, 1:01 p.m., https://twitter.com/Headspace/status/1108428244435550208?s=20&t=Wn513OFQjJ1CYuBS9K4Anw.

2   "16 Types of Meditation," Headspace, accessed October 14, 2022, https://www.headspace.com/meditation/techniques.

3   "16 Types of Meditation."

4   Dr. Swami Shankardev Saraswati, "Definitions of Yoga," Big Shakti, January 14, 2011, https://bigshakti.com/definitions-of-yoga/.

5   Shankardev Saraswati, "Definitions of Yoga."

6   Gwen Dittmar, "Breathwork: How to Tap into the Incredible Power of Breath," mbgmindfullness, February 16, 2020, https://www.mindbodygreen.com/articles/what-breathwork-is/.

7   Dittmar, "Breathwork."

8   Carol Dweck, *Mindset: The New Psychology of Success* (New York: Balantine Books, 2006), 4.

9   Simon Sinek, *Start with Why: How Great Leaders Inspire Everyone to Take Action* (New York: Portfolio, 2009), 73-74.

10 "'Pursuit of Happiness Is Fundamental Human Goal,' Minister of Bhutan Tells UN Assembly," United Nations, October 3, 2015, https://news.un.org/en/story/2015/10/511502-pursuit-happiness-fundamental-human-goal-minister-bhutan-tells-un-assembly/.

11   David A. Sbarra, Hillary L. Smith, and Matthias R. Mehl, "When Leaving Your Ex, Love Yourself: Observational Ratings of Self-Compassion Predict the Course of Emotional Recovery Following Marital Separation," *Psychological Science* 23, no. 3 (2012): 261–269, https://doi.org/10.1177/0956797611429466.

12   Seth Godin, "The Hierarchy of Success," *Seth's Blog*, September 14, 2019, https://seths.blog/2009/09/the-hierarchy-of-success/.

13   Edwin A. Locke and Gary P. Latham, "New Directions in Goal-Setting Theory," *Current Directions in Psychological Science* 15, no. 5 (2006): 265–268, https://doi.org/10.1111/j.1467-8721.2006.00449.x.

14   Barry J. Zimmerman, Albert Bandura, and Manuel Martinez-Pons, "Self-Motivation for Academic Attainment: The Role of Self-Efficacy Beliefs and Personal Goal Setting," *American Educational Research Association* 29, no. 3 (1992): 663–676, https://doi.org/10.3102/00028312029003663.

15   Jian Wang et al., "Neuropeptide Y in Relation to Carbohydrate Intake, Corticosterone and Dietary Obesity," *Brain Research* 802, no. 1–2 (1998): 75–88, https://doi.org/10.1016/S0006-8993(98)00551-4; Bernard Beck, "Neuropeptide Y in Normal Eating and in Genetic and Dietary-Induced Obesity," *Philosophical Transactions of the Royal Society B: Biological Sciences* 361, no. 1471 (2006): 1159–1185, https://doi.org/10.1098/rstb.2006.1855.

16   Clare Anderson and Charlotte R. Platten, "Sleep Deprivation Lowers Inhibition and Enhances Impulsivity to Negative Stimuli," *Behavioural Brain Research* 217, no. 2 (2011): 463–466, https://doi.org/10.1016/j.bbr.2010.09.020.

17   "Amygdala," Brain Made Simple, September 24, 2019, https://brainmadesimple.com/amygdala/.

18   Lisa Y. M. Chuah et al., "Sleep Deprivation and Interference by Emotional Distracters," *Sleep* 33, no. 10 (2010): 1305–1313, https://doi.org/10.1093/sleep/33.10.1305.

19   William D. S. Killgore, "Chapter 30 – Sleep Deprivation and Behavioral Risk-Taking," in *Modulation of Sleep by Obesity, Diabetes, Age, and Diet*, ed. Ronald Ross Watson (Cambridge, MA: Academic Press, 2015): 279–287, https://doi.org/10.1016/B978-0-12-420168-2.00030-2.

20   Christopher M. Barnes, "Sleep-Deprived People Are More Likely to Cheat," *Harvard Business Review*, May 31, 2013, https://hbr.org/2013/05/sleep-deprived-people-are-more-likely-to-cheat.

21   Sarah Hanson and Andy Jones, "Is There Evidence that Walking Groups Have Health Benefits? A Systematic Review and Meta-Analysis," *British Journal of Sports Medicine* 49, no. 11 (2015): 710–715, http://dx.doi.org/10.1136/bjsports-2014-094157.

22 J. C. Miller and Z. Krizan, "Walking Facilities Positive Affect (Even When Expecting the Opposite)," *Emotion* 16, no. 5 (2016): 775–785, https://doi.org/10.1037/a0040270.

23 Gregory N. Bratman, "Nature Experience Reduces Rumination and Subgenual Prefrontal Cortex Activation," *PNAS* 112, no. 28 (2015): 8567–8572, https://doi.org/10.1073/pnas.1510459112.

24 Kory Taylor and Elizabeth B. Jones, *Adult Dehydration* (Treasure Island, FL: StatPearls Publishing, 2022), https://www.ncbi.nlm.nih.gov/books/NBK555956/.

25 Jaecheol Moon and Gwanpyo Koh, "Clinical Evidence and Mechanisms of High-Protein Diet-Induced Weight Loss," *Journal of Obesity & Metabolic Syndrome* 29, no. 3 (2020): 166–173, https://doi.org/10.7570/jomes20028.

26 Douglas Paddon-Jones et al., "Protein, Weight Management, and Satiety," *The American Journal of Clinical Nutrition* 87, no. 5 (2008): 1558S–1561S, https://doi.org/10.1093/ajcn/87.5.1558s.

27 Anne-Marie Ravn et al., "Thermic Effect of a Meal and Appetite in Adults: An Individual Participant Data Meta-Analysis of Meal-Test Trials," *Food & Nutrition Research* 57 (2013), https://doi.org/10.3402/fnr.v57i0.19676.

28 Dominik H. Pesta and Varman T. Samuel, "A High-Protein Diet for Reducing Body Fat: Mechanisms and Possible Caveats," *Nutrition & Metabolism* 11, no. 53 (2014), https://doi.org/10.1186/1743-7075-11-53.

29 Pesta and Samuel, "High-Protein Diet."

30 Heather J. Leidy, "Increased Dietary Protein as a Dietary Strategy to Prevent and/or Treat Obesity," *Missouri Medicine* 111, no. 1 (January–February 2014): 54–58, https://www.omagdigital.com/publication/?m=11307&i=197433&p=56&ver=html5

31 M. S. Westerterp-Plantenga et al., "High Protein Intake Sustains Weight Maintenance After Body Weight Loss in Humans," *International Journal Obesity* 28 (2004): 57–64, https://doi.org/10.1038/sj.ijo.0802461.

32 Petra Stiegler and Adam Cunliffe, "The Role of Diet and Exercise for the Maintenance of Fat-Free Mass and Resting Metabolic Rate During Weight Loss," *Sports Medicine* 36 (2006): 239–262, https://doi.org/10.2165/00007256-200636030-00005.

33 Check out bodzii.com/blog for many high-protein recipes to help hit protein targets.

34 Dweck, *Mindset*.

Manufactured by Amazon.ca
Bolton, ON

32047794R00102